Weightless

Weightless

A DOCTOR'S GUIDE TO
WEIGHT-LOSS MEDICATIONS,
SUSTAINABLE RESULTS AND
THE HEALTH YOU DESERVE

Dr Rocio Salas-Whalen
Foreword by Dr Mary Claire Haver

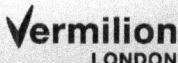

Vermilion
LONDON

VERMILION

UK | USA | Canada | Ireland | Australia
India | New Zealand | South Africa

Vermilion is part of the Penguin Random House group of companies
whose addresses can be found at global.penguinrandomhouse.com

Penguin Random House UK,
One Embassy Gardens, 8 Viaduct Gardens, London SW11 7BW

penguin.co.uk
global.penguinrandomhouse.com

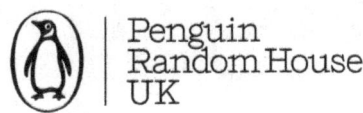

First published by Rodale Books in 2026
This edition published by Vermilion in 2026

2

Copyright © Rocio Salas-Whalen 2026
The moral right of the author has been asserted.

Penguin Random House values and supports copyright. Copyright fuels creativity, encourages diverse voices, promotes freedom of expression and supports a vibrant culture. Thank you for purchasing an authorised edition of this book and for respecting intellectual property laws by not reproducing, scanning or distributing any part of it by any means without permission. You are supporting authors and enabling Penguin Random House to continue to publish books for everyone. No part of this book may be used or reproduced in any manner for the purpose of training artificial intelligence technologies or systems. In accordance with Article 4(3) of the DSM Directive 2019/790, Penguin Random House expressly reserves this work from the text and data mining exception.

Typeset by Six Red Marbles UK, Thetford, Norfolk
Part-opening art by Kindlena/Shutterstock
Text box background art by BK_graphic/Shutterstock
Book design by Lorie Pagnozzi

Printed and bound in Great Britain by Clays Ltd, Elcograf S.p.A.

The authorised representative in the EEA is Penguin Random House Ireland,
Morrison Chambers, 32 Nassau Street, Dublin D02 YH68

A CIP catalogue record for this book is available from the British Library

Hardback ISBN 9781785046339
Trade Paperback ISBN 9781785046346

Penguin Random House is committed to a sustainable future
for our business, our readers and our planet. This book is made
from Forest Stewardship Council® certified paper.

To Isabel and Lucia: I will always be here for you, even in the pages of this book.

To my reader: You deserve quality care, real support, and honest guidance. Know that I wrote this book FOR YOU.

Contents

Foreword xi
Introduction xiii

Part I: The Road Ahead

CHAPTER 1
Rethinking Obesity: What We Got Wrong 3

CHAPTER 2
Enter GLP-1s: A New Era of Weight Management 29

CHAPTER 3
Are GLP-1s Right for You?: Evaluating Your Candidacy and Risks 54

CHAPTER 4
The Road Starts Here: Finding the Right Provider and Getting Your Prescription 76

Part II: Your Life-Changing Journey Begins

CHAPTER 5
Your GLP-1 Journey: What to Expect 101

CHAPTER 6
Staying on Course: Your GPS for Progress 127

CHAPTER 7
Titration and Troubleshooting: Adjusting Your Dose and Navigating Side Effects 157

Part III: Life After GLP-1s

CHAPTER 8
Maintaining Your Weight: Strategies for Sustained Success 181

CHAPTER 9
After the Transformation: Facing Yourself and the World 203

A Final Word 223

Protein Cheat Sheet 228
First Appointment Checklist 230
Follow-up Appointment Checklist 232
Acknowledgments 235
Notes 239
Index 253

DISCLAIMER

The information in this book has been compiled as general guidance on weight loss and obesity medicine, but is not a substitute and not to be relied on for medical, healthcare, pharmaceutical or other professional advice. Please consult your GP or medical practitioner before changing, stopping or starting any medical treatment or using GLP-1 medications. So far as the author is aware the information given is correct and up to date as at October 2025. Practice, laws and regulations all change, and the reader should obtain up-to-date professional advice on any such issues. The author and publishers disclaim, as far as the law allows, any liability arising directly or indirectly from the use, or misuse, of the information contained in this book.

Foreword

There are few moments in medicine when you can feel the ground shifting beneath your feet, when something long accepted as "just the way things are" suddenly cracks open, revealing a new truth. A better truth. One that reclaims hope, possibility, and dignity for patients who have been misunderstood for far too long.

The publication of this book, *Weightless*, marks one of those moments.

I'll be honest: When I first heard about GLP-1s being used for weight loss, I was skeptical. I was untrained in obesity medicine, underinformed, and hesitant to embrace what felt like a trend. But then Dr. Rocio Salas-Whalen changed everything for me. She figuratively held my hand, walked me through the science, and helped me understand the nuance. Because of her, I gained the confidence to incorporate GLP-1 therapy into my own practice—and I've seen firsthand how life-changing it can be when used responsibly, ethically, and with compassion.

I have known Rocio for years—as a colleague, a friend, and a physician whose expertise is matched only by her empathy. What you hold in your hands is not just a guide to GLP-1 medications; it is a corrective to decades of stigma, misinformation, and oversimplified narratives about obesity. It is the book we have needed for a very long time.

Weightless reframes obesity as the chronic, complex condition it truly is—not a willpower problem but a medical one. With clarity and care, Dr. Salas-Whalen offers readers the tools to understand their bodies, navigate treatment options, and reclaim control over their health journeys. This book is rigorous, compassionate, and deeply validating.

If you've felt dismissed, defeated, or confused by the conversation around weight, let this book be your antidote. It's time for a new conversation—one rooted in science, empathy, and empowerment.

Welcome to the weightless future. Let's begin.

—Mary Claire Haver, MD
Author of *The New Menopause* and *The Galveston Diet*

Introduction

First, an Apology

I can't tell you how happy I am that you picked up this book. This means that you're on a GLP-1 medication, you are a family member or friend of someone taking one, or you might be considering using one for weight management. GLP-1 therapy will be the first step toward feeling better—physically, mentally, and emotionally. But before we go any further, I want to say something I don't think patients hear nearly enough: I'm sorry.

This is an apology letter to anyone who has struggled with weight. Whether you've carried the burden of obesity your entire life, fought constantly to lose those last ten or twenty pounds, cycled through endless diets, or battled persistent food thoughts, I'm writing this book for you. And the first thing I want to do is apologize on behalf of the medical community.

For too long, we approached chronic conditions such as obesity as "willpower problems" or moral failings. We sent patients home with oversimplified advice about "calories in, calories out," and when the numbers on their scales didn't go down, we chalked it up to noncompliance. We treated the symptoms but did nothing to treat the disease because we didn't fully understand it as a medical condition. In the process, we caused our patients struggling with obesity and weight loss to become intensely distrustful of healthcare providers.

It wasn't until recently that we began to look at weight management in a new light. GLP-1s flooded the market on the heels of the covid pandemic. This newfound attention has both upsides and downsides. The increased aid, research, treatment, and evolving mindsets about obesity are definite positives. But the rapid bandwagon-style adoption of these drugs—without proper assessment, monitoring, or strategic approaches—has led to serious issues. Many doctors, often with little experience with weight management, are tossing prescriptions to patients without offering even the most basic guidance on how to use them effectively or avoid serious side effects such as muscle loss. After wrongly telling patients for years that their weight problems were their fault, doctors are suddenly offering a "miracle drug" to solve a multifaceted health problem. Many of them haven't been studying weight management for the last dozen years, so while they struggle to catch up to the specialists who have, patients are left to wade through this new world on their own. The medical community is waking up and wants to help, but in a lot of cases, patients are still being set up to fail. While GLP-1s are revolutionary, they're just one piece of this complex puzzle. I'm here to put it all together for you.

Let Me Introduce Myself

I'm Rocio Salas-Whalen, a board-certified physician who specializes in obesity medicine and endocrinology. As a little girl growing up in Mexico, I always knew exactly what I wanted to do: I wanted to be a doctor. It was never a question of what I wanted to be when I grew up; it was a matter of when and how.

My determination to become a doctor grew even fiercer when my father was diagnosed with type 2 diabetes while I was in medical school. His diagnosis was terrifying to me. I'd always known that my grandfather had passed away from the disease before I was born. Diabetes was the first major health issue I'd ever heard of, and it felt like a specter that lurked around every corner. In Mexico, it's the third leading cause of death. By my third year in medical school, I knew for certain that endocrinology was the right path for me. I didn't want to just treat diseases such as diabetes, but prevent them from happening. I wanted to help patients make lasting lifestyle changes to reduce their risk.

In 2006, when I was a resident doing my endocrinology rotation, I had the privilege of attending a grand rounds presentation by Dr. John Eng, a pioneer in the development of GLP-1 medications (you'll learn more about him and his discoveries in chapter 2). At that point, I was already extremely interested in metabolic health, so to me, it was a once-in-a-lifetime moment, one that changed how I practiced medicine. I was blown away by his research and insights. At the time, GLP-1s were very new, but they clearly had immense potential. I immediately recognized that they were going to be a game changer in our treatment of metabolic conditions such as diabetes and maybe even obesity.

After completing my fellowship, I was excited to discover that there was a new medical specialty specifically for obesity. I immediately knew that I wanted to become board certified in obesity medicine to deepen my knowledge of and background in weight management.

In 2010, I was finally done with training and moved into practicing. At the clinic where I worked, I began prescribing Byetta, one of the first GLP-1 medications, as soon as I was able to. I couldn't wait to see how those medications could change lives. The results my patients achieved with GLP-1s, even in those early days, made me a firm believer in the power of these treatments. And over the years, they've been getting better—more effective and with fewer side effects. What was once a revolutionary treatment has now become a common solution for managing obesity and metabolic conditions.

Today, I have a thriving practice in New York City and continue to prescribe the latest versions of GLP-1 medications as they evolve. I've been thrilled to watch the treatment work its way into the mainstream and help thousands throughout the country and the world—and I've even taken them myself during two different periods of my life! (I'll share more about one of these experiences in chapter 3.)

That said, to most people, these medications are a new frontier. Many providers don't know how to match patients with the right GLP-1 for their needs; others are not prescribing the correct dosage. Most patients are not getting the nutritional or mental health support they need alongside GLP-1 treatment. Unfortunately, I'm just one person—but it shouldn't just be a privileged few who get help at my Park Avenue office. So I've written this book to mirror the experience I offer my patients as best I can.

As one of the few endocrinologists in the world who has been specializing in obesity medicine since the advent of GLP-1 treatment, I've listened to the testimonials of thousands of patients. I have a unique body of knowledge, and I want to disseminate this information to as many people as possible. There aren't enough experienced doctors, but hopefully, with this book, there will be well-informed patients.

What's Ahead?

In the pages that follow, I will take you on a comprehensive health journey that begins before you take your first dose. I'll be your guide as you undergo the process of losing weight and navigate life after you achieve your weight loss goals. We'll discuss everything you need to know about GLP-1 medications: how they work, their side effects, how to preserve muscle and get enough protein, lifestyle changes to make, and more. Along the way, I'll share testimonials from real patients of mine who share their experiences with GLP-1 therapy and how some of them navigated the common obstacles in their journeys.

Each of these chapters is designed to build on the last to give you a complete foundation for your GLP-1 journey. If you ever need to revisit a topic, it's not a step backward; it's part of learning. Right now, you have access to knowledge—real, practical knowledge that's yours to keep and return to any time you need support or clarity.

Throughout this book, you'll notice that I use person-first language when referring to people with obesity or related health conditions. That means you'll see phrases such as "a patient with obesity" instead of "an obese patient" and "a person with overweight" instead of "an overweight person."

This isn't just a matter of semantics. It's very important to me always to frame obesity as a medical condition, never as a personal failing or defining trait. Language matters, and how we talk about health can shape how we think about it. When we put the person before the diagnosis, we're not blaming the patient; we're reinforcing a core belief of this book: *You are not your weight.*

As a doctor, I advocate for every one of my patients to be treated with compassion and respect; of course, I'm going to do the same for you readers.

Ultimately, I want this book to serve as a comprehensive companion for you. I think of it as a veritable love letter to my patients over the years, and for everyone who reads it, it is my way of saying **"You are not alone, and you are not doing this alone."** You have research-based support, a group of people who have been where you are, and, most important, a hand to hold while you walk into the increasingly bright future on the path to better health.

Even more important, I hope that this book helps you feel what the title promises: weightless. Not just with your body but also with your thoughts and feelings. Weightless of shame, guilt, and the belief that you failed because the standard advice failed you. Weightless of a stigma by a culture that never fully saw you. Weightless of the burden of carrying it all every day.

With the help of GLP-1 therapy and the guidance you'll find in these pages, I hope you can begin to let some of that weight go. I hope you'll begin to feel lighter—and not just physically but emotionally and psychologically. I hope you'll begin to imagine a life where your health no longer feels like a battle and your worth isn't—and never has been—up for debate. That's what weightless means to me. I hope that by the end of this book, it will mean something powerful to you, too.

Sincerely,
Dr. Rocio Salas-Whalen

PART I
The Road Ahead

CHAPTER 1

Rethinking Obesity: What We Got Wrong

There is one patient consultation that has stayed with me over the years. The patient was fifty-one years old, successful in his career, polite, thoughtful—and clearly uneasy the moment he stepped into my office. When I asked what had brought him in, he explained that he had tried everything: dieting, fasting, overexercising. He had lost weight many times but always gained it back. He said, "I guess I'm just not trying hard enough, but I just don't know what else to do."

I shook my head and told him, "Obesity is not your fault."

I explained what we now understand about obesity: that it's not just about what you eat or how much you move; it's about hormones, genetics, the brain, the gut, and many other factors outside of willpower. And then something unexpected happened. There was a visible shift; I watched the tension in his shoulders ease as his emotional burden was lifted. He started to cry. For the first time, he heard that he hadn't failed. He felt the validation that what he was up against wasn't a personal flaw but a medical condition.

And I hadn't even told him the best part yet: *There was something we could do about it.*

When I see a reaction like that, it makes me want to share everything I've learned about obesity with everyone—and repeat it over and over. In this chapter, you'll learn what's going on "behind the scenes of the body" and the reasons behind weight gain in cases like my patient's—and maybe yours, even if you don't identify with the term *obesity*.

Whether or not you've been formally diagnosed with obesity, this is a crucial chapter to help you understand your body and its treatment in a whole new way. If you're someone with excess weight who is considering taking a GLP-1 medication—or even just trying to better understand why your body holds on to weight despite all your efforts—read on.

In the pages ahead, we'll pull back the curtain on what obesity actually is: not a character flaw but a disease influenced by many aspects of our biology and environment. I share this information not to lecture you but to make your experience with GLP-1 therapy more effective, more comprehensive, and ultimately more empowering. I want you to understand that this treatment is informed by real people and real life. Along the way, you'll also begin to see the full picture of obesity—one grounded in science, not bias.

There's much to learn ahead, but just as important, there's much to unlearn.

Understanding Obesity

In medicine, there is a commonly accepted idea that within the patient/doctor dynamic, it is only the patient who needs to learn. This couldn't be further from the truth, and I am proof of this. In my opinion, a physician who is not learning is a physician who is not listening to their patients.

For decades, medical professionals have been taught to approach obesity as a simple math problem: Eat less, exercise more. This advice was repeated in exam rooms, public health campaigns, and weight loss programs. And because it was presented as a straightforward solution, it also carried an unspoken assumption: If a patient wasn't losing weight, it must have been due to a lack of effort, discipline, or willpower.

But if this approach truly worked, why did obesity rates continue to rise? Why do millions of people—many of whom have followed every diet, exercise plan, and medical recommendation—still find themselves struggling with their weight? The answer: It's not because patients aren't trying but because this approach to treating obesity is fundamentally flawed.

To fully grasp the scope of this issue, let's step back and examine the bigger picture. The statistics on obesity tell a story—one that makes it clear that obesity isn't just a personal challenge but a global public health emergency.

The Landscape of Obesity: A Global and National Crisis

Obesity is defined as the abnormal or excessive expansion of adipose tissue. It is a complex disease that affects nearly half of all U.S. adults, and its prevalence is increasing worldwide.

According to the World Health Organization (WHO), worldwide obesity rates have nearly tripled since 1975. Nearly every developed nation has experienced an increase in obesity prevalence. The United States has been at the forefront of this crisis; I'm sure it's no surprise to you that our obesity rate has been rising at an alarming pace. In 1962, only 13 percent of U.S. adults were classified as having obesity. By 1999, that number had skyrocketed to 30.5 percent. By 2020, obesity affected 41.9 percent of

U.S. adults. And today, nearly one in five children in the United States lives with obesity.

At the current trajectory, nearly half of U.S. adults will be classified as having obesity in the next decade. But this is not just an American problem; it's a global phenomenon. Countries around the world, from the United Kingdom to China, are experiencing rising obesity rates.

What changed? Just a few generations ago, obesity was far less common. People moved more, food was less processed, and portion sizes were smaller. But today's world looks different. The rise of ultraprocessed foods has made calorie-dense, nutrient-poor options more accessible and affordable than ever before. Sedentary lifestyles have become the norm, with more jobs shifting to office work and many people working remotely. Cities are designed for cars instead of pedestrians, and there are fewer opportunities for physical activity built into daily life. Stress, poor sleep, and environmental factors have contributed to weight gain in ways that weren't as prevalent in previous generations. The result? A public health crisis that affects every aspect of society.

Obesity is not just about physical appearance or weight; it is directly linked to serious chronic diseases. Individuals with obesity are at higher risk of developing type 2 diabetes, heart disease, stroke, and more than thirteen obesity-related cancers. Because it increases the risk of these diseases, it can shorten lifespan significantly, making it one of the most notable modifiable risk factors for early death. But the impact goes beyond physical health; obesity is also tied to higher rates of depression and anxiety and increases the likelihood of experiencing social stigma, creating a vicious cycle that makes weight management even more difficult.

Obesity is not a simple condition, and it is certainly not just a result of individual lifestyle choices. If personal effort alone were enough, we would have seen a decline in obesity rates, not a continued surge. This crisis is not the result of individual failures; it is the result of a systemic misunderstanding of obesity within the medical community and beyond.

But what if we could change this trajectory? Imagine a world where individuals could live longer, healthier lives, where the healthcare system wasn't overwhelmed by preventable diseases, and where people had the energy, confidence, and physical well-being to fully engage in their lives. What if instead of reacting to obesity by shrugging our shoulders, we addressed it as a treatable medical condition?

Beyond Willpower: The Real Causes of Excess Fat Tissue

Throughout the many years of my career, I have seen thousands of patients. Each one of them has taught me something about this varied and persistent disease. What I believed at the start of my practice is not what I believe today. Over time, I have amassed an entirely new body of knowledge—not from textbooks but from the patients themselves. But before I could learn from them, I had to unlearn much of what I was taught.

For decades, we told patients that obesity and overweight were a personal problem—a matter of willpower, discipline, and self-control. Patients who struggled with their weight were told the same thing over and over: *Eat less. Move more. Try harder. Repeat.*

When a patient who had overweight or obesity would tell us that they followed the recommendations but did not lose weight, we did the worst thing possible: *We didn't believe them.* If after several appointments the patient's weight seemed static or even increased, then either the doctor or the patient, sometimes both of them, would come to see that lack of progress as an impossible hurdle to overcome—and simply stop talking about it. We would instead turn to treating the symptoms of obesity because, for them, we did have medications that provided results. In the medical community, conventional wisdom told us that that was the best we could do.

It wasn't until I started seeing patients with obesity five days a week, eight hours a day, that I finally learned something new—something that defied what I'd been taught in medical school: Our patients *were* listening to us.

Not only did they obviously understand the simple "calories in, calories out" formula, but they were following it—and going above and beyond. They counted calories, cut carbs, avoided fats, and exercised relentlessly. They'd tried it all: fasting, juice cleanses, Atkins, keto, paleo, SlimFast, Weight Watchers. (A Google search will show you that there are *hundreds* of weight loss diets out there, and these patients are more familiar with them than anyone else.) They'd exhausted exercise programs and trainers. Some had spent thousands of dollars on so-called fat camps with only temporary success. This happened for both people who had struggled with weight for their entire lives and those who had experienced weight gain after hitting a certain age or a certain life event (such as pregnancy, menopause, or illness).

Even for the people who drastically transformed their habits, their results were not the expected ones and were nonlasting. Our patients were doing exactly what we told them to do. But the weight wouldn't come off, no matter what they did. When they'd report this back to us, we'd tell them again: *Eat even less. Move even more. Try harder.* It's no surprise that patients who struggle to manage their weight grow to dislike doctors.

And you know what? I can't blame them. We, the medical community, had failed them, and we had some things to change.

Obesity was recognized as a disease in 1948 by the World Health Organization (WHO)—but it wasn't until 2013 that the American Medical Association (AMA) formally classified it as a *chronic, multifactorial* disease. This may sound like a minor distinction, but it reflected a major shift in medical understanding—one that forced us doctors to rethink the way we approached its treatment.

When we talk about multifactorial chronic diseases, we think of type 2 diabetes, chronic hypertension, and chronic hyperlipidemia. We know that lifestyle can affect them, but we also recognize them as medical conditions influenced by a complex web of factors, many of which patients have little control over. The same applies to obesity.

We spent decades telling patients that obesity was a behavioral issue, but it is a medical condition influenced by a range of biological, hormonal, genetic, and environmental factors.

HOLLY'S STORY

Since I was a young girl, weight loss was emphasized in every aspect of my life. What I ate and how I ate it was a constant topic of conversation with family. The word *fat* was used so often, it became a part of my daily vocabulary. I became so self-conscious and constantly felt uncomfortable in my own skin.

I spent years becoming a professional dieter, an expert exerciser, and a pursuer of all things healthy; my goal was to be fit and pleasing to everyone around me. In all that time, with all that effort, I never attained my "perfect weight." I cycled through weight loss and regain over and over again. I tried it all—every diet and exercise program out there: FA, Weight

Watchers, Jenny Craig, Special K, the cabbage diet, intermittent fasting, cleanses, boot camps, HIIT workouts, group exercises, walking four to six miles a day.

By forty-five, I was really suffering. The food noise was at an all-time high. I was in a tough place—dealing with perimenopause and having children later in life. Five more years went by before real conversations about getting help started to gain traction.

Then I heard Dr. Salas-Whalen speak, and I saw in her such a sincere and compassionate physician. For the first time, I wondered: Could I have been misled about weight? Everything she was saying was backed by scientific studies. I called and made an appointment.

Last May, my life instantly changed—and that's not an exaggeration. The medication calmed me almost immediately. I felt grounded. I lost forty-four pounds gradually and only lost one pound of muscle. It was a slow process, and I felt cared for and supported.

Now I have so much hope. It feels like I am finally living. My prayer is for others to realize that we've been given a great gift to help in the battle against obesity.

The Factors Behind Obesity and Excess Weight

Whether you've been diagnosed with obesity or just know you're carrying extra weight that you can't seem to lose, the same root causes often apply. In the next section, we'll explore the six major contributors to weight gain and weight retention. These factors go far beyond "calories in, calories out." Understanding them will help explain what's going on behind the scenes in your body and help you understand how to get the most out of your GLP-1 treatment.

1. Genes and Epigenetic Changes

Obesity is profoundly influenced by both genetic and epigenetic factors. Some people are biologically predisposed to gain weight more easily than others due to genetic inheritance and epigenetic modifications that shape their metabolism, appetite, and fat storage. Understanding these mechanisms can help us understand the underlying weight management challenges that many face.

Genes: How Your DNA Shapes Your Weight

Your genetics are the blueprint that determines how your body responds to food, hunger signals, and fat storage. If you have a family history of obesity, your body may be biologically wired in ways that make weight regulation more difficult. Some people are born with a higher risk of obesity; it's a matter of inherited biology. For example, there are variations in genes that impact appetite regulation, fat storage, and metabolism, such as FTO, MC4R, and LEPR genes. Genetic traits that increase the chance of developing a preference for highly palatable, calorie-dense foods can be passed down to the next generation.

How Your Genes May Increase the Risk of Obesity
- **You burn fewer calories at rest,** making weight gain more likely.
- **You have a blunted satiety response;** you don't feel full after eating until later, leading to overeating.
- **There are differences in your brain's reward system,** leading to more intense cravings for high-calorie foods.
- **You have a harder time losing weight** than others do, even when following the same diet and exercise plan.

Epigenetics: How Your Environment Modifies Genetic Expression

While your genes are fixed at birth, your lifestyle and environment can lead to changes in your gene expression, affecting whether certain genes are turned off or on. These modifications are known as epigenetic changes.

Epigenetics explains why two people who grew up with different environments, diets, and early-life conditions may experience different weight outcomes, despite having the same genetic predisposition for obesity. Epigenetic changes can influence people even before birth. We know that parents' weight at preconception—yes, *preconception*—can determine the weight of their future offspring.

Epigenetic Factors That Influence Obesity

- **Parental weight/diet before conception:** Both parents' weight and nutrition prior to conception can alter gene expression in offspring, increasing the child's obesity risk.
- **In utero environment:** A fetus exposed to poor maternal nutrition, stress, or excess weight gain during pregnancy is more likely to have a body that favors fat storage and develops insulin resistance.
- **Early-childhood diet:** High consumption of ultraprocessed foods in infancy and early childhood can cause epigenetic changes that lead to lifelong obesity risk.
- **Transgenerational trauma and stress exposure:** The high stress experienced by previous generations due to events such as famine, economic hardship, or traumatic events can epigenetically alter their offspring's stress responses, affecting their fat retention and metabolism.
- **Nutrient deficiencies:** Lack of key nutrients during fetal development (such as folate and omega-3 fats) can alter metabolic pathways.

2. Your Hormones

Hormones are the body's chemical messengers; they regulate hunger, metabolism, fat storage, and energy use. Disruptions in hormonal balance can make weight gain more likely and weight loss more difficult, even with lifestyle changes.

Key Hormones That Influence Obesity
- **Insulin:** Insulin is responsible for glucose uptake and fat storage. When a person's insulin level is chronically elevated (as with insulin resistance), the body is more likely to store fat instead of burning it. Obesity and insulin resistance create a vicious cycle: Excess fat makes cells more resistant to insulin, and the pancreas compensates by producing more insulin, further promoting fat storage. Conditions linked to insulin dysfunction include metabolic syndrome (a cluster of conditions that together raise the risk of heart disease and diabetes) and prediabetes/type 2 diabetes.
- **Leptin:** Leptin is produced by fat cells, and it signals the brain when the body has stored enough energy. Leptin resistance occurs when the brain no longer responds to leptin's signal, leading to increased hunger and decreased energy expenditure. People with obesity often have a high leptin level, yet their body fails to recognize the signals to stop eating.
- **Ghrelin:** Ghrelin is secreted in the stomach and stimulates appetite, especially before meals. Normally, a person's ghrelin level drops after eating, but in some individuals, it remains elevated, leading to persistent hunger and overeating.
- **Cortisol:** Cortisol is the body's main stress hormone, released by the adrenal glands. A chronically high cortisol level promotes fat storage, especially in the abdominal area.

- **Estrogen:** Estrogen influences where fat is stored—for example, around the hips and thighs versus the abdomen. A drop in estrogen level during menopause contributes to central (abdominal) weight gain.
- **Testosterone:** A low testosterone level in both men and women can contribute to increased fat mass and reduced muscle mass, making weight regulation more difficult.
- **Thyroid hormones (T3 and T4):** These hormones regulate metabolism. In hypothyroidism (underactive thyroid), the metabolic rate slows down, which can contribute to weight gain.
- **Peptide YY (PYY) and GLP-1:** These gut hormones help promote satiety (feeling full). Levels of PYY and GLP-1 are often lower in individuals with obesity, which may contribute to overeating.

Hormonal Conditions That Can Cause Weight Gain
- **Insulin resistance:** Insulin resistance is a metabolic condition in which the body's cells become less responsive to the action of insulin, a hormone produced by the pancreas that helps regulate the blood glucose level by facilitating the uptake of glucose into cells for energy.

    When insulin resistance occurs, the body compensates by producing more insulin (hyperinsulinemia) to maintain a normal blood glucose level. Over time, this compensatory mechanism can fail, leading to elevated blood sugar, increased fat storage (particularly visceral fat), and a cascade of metabolic dysfunctions.
- **Polycystic ovarian syndrome (PCOS):** PCOS is one of the most common—and unfortunately most overlooked—hormonal disorders in women. It is strongly associated with insulin resistance and an elevated insulin level (hyperinsulinemia), both of which contribute to increased visceral fat, which, in turn, promotes the conversion

of estradiol (a form of estrogen) into testosterone. An elevated testosterone level can disrupt the menstrual cycle, causing irregular periods and fertility issues. The hormonal imbalance not only affects reproductive health but also makes weight loss more difficult. Other contributing symptoms include chronic inflammation, which exacerbates insulin resistance, contributing to a vicious cycle that makes PCOS challenging to manage.

- **Hypothyroidism:** The thyroid regulates metabolism, body temperature, and energy level. Hypothyroidism (an underactive thyroid) leads to slowed metabolism, weight gain, and fatigue. Common symptoms of thyroid-related weight gain include a sluggish metabolism (burning fewer calories at rest), fluid retention and bloating, and difficulty losing weight despite diet and exercise.

- **Cushing's syndrome/disease:** This condition is caused by chronic excess cortisol, either from internal overproduction (e.g., by adrenal or pituitary tumors) or the long-term use of corticosteroids. Cushing's syndrome causes obesity because excess cortisol increases fat storage, especially in the abdomen, face, and upper back. It also promotes insulin resistance, which leads to higher blood sugar and more fat storage. It breaks down muscle, decreasing metabolism and physical strength. Together, these effects shift the body toward storing fat instead of burning it, especially in the central body.

- **Low testosterone:** Low testosterone can occur in both men and women. It leads to decreased muscle mass and increased fat mass. It is often overlooked, especially in aging adults.

Life Stages and Hormonal Shifts That Influence Weight

- **Pregnancy and postpartum weight retention:** During pregnancy, some women develop increased insulin resistance, a condition known as gestational diabetes, which can make postpartum weight retention more likely. Weight gain is also more likely during the postpartum period because of an elevated cortisol level due to stress, sleep deprivation, and the demands of caring for a newborn. While some women experience weight loss while breastfeeding, others may have a reduced metabolic rate, making it more difficult to shed excess weight gained during pregnancy.

- **Perimenopause and menopause:** As the estrogen level declines during menopause, fat distribution shifts, leading to increased abdominal fat storage. A decrease in estrogen is also associated with a slower metabolism, making weight management more challenging. A lower estrogen level contributes to increased insulin resistance, which can make the body more prone to storing excess fat. Due to changes in estrogen level, postmenopausal women face a higher risk of developing metabolic conditions, including diabetes and cardiovascular disease.

3. Your Environment

While our individual biology plays a powerful role in how our bodies gain and store weight, our surroundings can also either support or sabotage our health. From the chemicals we're exposed to to how our neighborhoods are built, our environment quietly but profoundly influences factors that promote weight gain.

The Industrialized Food System: Engineered for Overconsumption

It's nearly impossible to walk into a grocery store, gas station, or even pharmacy without encountering shelves of highly processed, hyperpalatable foods. These foods are filled with refined sugars, saturated fats, and artificial additives—and they're designed to override your natural hunger and fullness signals, leading to overeating and weight gain.

Ultraprocessed foods now make up more than 50 percent of the average American's diet. These foods are intentionally addictive, triggering the release of dopamine in our brain, making us crave more. The food industry spends billions of dollars on marketing each year to encourage their consumption, often targeting children and vulnerable populations.

Big Agriculture and the food industry profit from a population hooked on calorie-dense, nutritionally poor foods. Much like the way the tobacco industry downplayed the risks of smoking for decades, food corporations have strategically marketed processed foods while dismissing their direct role in the obesity epidemic.

Your Emotional and Social Environment

For many people, the most powerful environmental influences are the ones we carry inside us. They're embedded in our physiology and shaped by our lived experience. The factors influencing the emotional and social environments we grow up in—our earliest relationships, our chronic stressors, and even our community's collective history—can all shape the way our bodies regulate weight.

Trauma and Your Body

For some people, the roots of weight gain trace back to their early life. Adverse childhood experiences (ACEs), such as abuse, neglect, or household instability, are strongly linked to obesity in adulthood. The more ACEs a person experiences, the higher their risk of having obesity. These early stressors can disrupt the body's stress response system, keeping the cortisol level elevated and promoting fat storage, particularly around the abdomen.

Even when trauma isn't dramatic or obvious, its effects can have a deep impact. Ongoing emotional stress, invalidation, or fear during critical periods of development can rewire the brain's reward system. This rewiring can look different for each person, but for many people, it makes high-fat, high-sugar foods more appealing and comforting. Eating becomes a form of self-soothing, creating a behavior that is learned early and reinforced over time.

Generational Trauma
Sometimes the influences on our weight go back further than we realize. Families often carry more than just shared genes; they carry the imprint of past hardship, stress, or trauma. These patterns, passed down through generations, can shape our relationship with food, our stress responses, and the way our bodies store fat. You might not know the full details of your grandparents' lives, but if they lived through war, poverty, systemic oppression, or chronic stress, that legacy may have reached you—not just emotionally but through epigenic changes, as discussed earlier. What looks like a personal weight struggle is often the echo of much older survival adaptations.

Chronic Stress and Marginalization: The Invisible Burden
Living with ongoing stress—especially when it stems from systemic issues such as discrimination, financial insecurity, or social exclusion—can take a profound toll on the body. Chronic stress keeps the body's alarm system activated, elevating cortisol and increasing fat storage over time. Entire communities carry the health consequences of long-term marginalization. These invisible burdens often go unrecognized in medical settings, yet they're central to the lived experience of many patients.

Endocrine Disruptors: Chemicals That Alter Metabolism

Beyond what we eat, our environment is filled with chemicals that affect the way our bodies regulate weight. Endocrine-disrupting chemicals (EDCs) are found in plastics, pesticides, and even personal care products. They mimic hormones such as estrogen and disrupt your natural metabolic processes, making weight gain more likely. Examples of EDCs include BPAs, parabens, and some pesticides and herbicides. These chemicals don't just affect individuals; they impact entire populations, influencing obesity rates across generations.

Sedentary Lifestyles: Fewer Opportunities for Daily Movement

As briefly touched upon above, the decline in physical activity over the past few decades is not just a population getting "lazier"; it has been driven largely by shifts in work culture, urban planning, and technological advancements. The rise of desk jobs and remote work means that many of us spend entire days sitting, with fewer opportunities for natural movement. Car-dependent cities lead us to walk less, while automation and convenience technologies have replaced many daily activities that once required a bit, for example Instacart and Taskrabbit, of physical effort. Even people who make a conscious effort to stay active still operate within an environment that systematically requires less and less daily movement, making weight gain more likely.

4. Aging and Metabolic Changes

As we age, maintaining a healthy weight becomes increasingly difficult—not due to lack of effort but because of biological changes in metabolism, muscle mass, and hormone regulation.

While many people assume that weight gain is inevitable with age, the reality is that aging itself changes the way our bodies process energy, store fat, and regulate hunger signals.

Metabolic Slowdown: Why We Burn Fewer Calories as We Age

One of the biggest contributors to age-related weight gain is the natural decline in metabolic rate. The body's basal metabolic rate (BMR), the number of calories burned at rest, decreases by approximately 1 to 2 percent per decade after age twenty. This means that even if a person maintains the same diet and activity level, they may gradually gain weight because their body is burning fewer calories than before.

Several factors contribute to this metabolic slowdown:
- **Decreased mitochondrial efficiency:** The body's cells become less efficient at converting food into energy.
- **Reduced thyroid hormone activity:** As people age, their thyroid function can decline, slowing their metabolism.
- **Changes in insulin sensitivity:** Older adults often become more insulin resistant, which increases their fat storage, particularly in the abdomen.

Muscle Loss (Sarcopenia): The Silent Driver of Weight Gain

Aging is also associated with progressive muscle loss, known as sarcopenia. After age thirty, adults lose 3 to 8 percent of their muscle mass per decade, and this process accelerates after age sixty. Since muscle is more metabolically active than fat, a loss of muscle means that the body burns fewer calories while at rest, making weight gain more likely. Factors contributing to sarcopenia include:
- **Hormonal changes** (declines in testosterone, estrogen, and growth hormone)

- Reduced physical activity (especially strength training)
- Lower protein intake (many older adults eat fewer protein-rich foods)

Muscle loss doesn't just contribute to weight gain; it also reduces mobility, increases the risk of falling, and weakens overall metabolic health. But we'll talk a lot more about muscle loss (and how to prevent it!) in chapter 6.

5. Medications

For many people, weight gain isn't just about diet and exercise; it's about their medications. We now know that many commonly prescribed drugs directly contribute to weight gain. Unfortunately, patients are often not informed of this side effect, leaving them frustrated when they see the scale creeping up despite their making lifestyle changes. Certain medications can promote weight gain by:

- **Increasing appetite:** Some drugs stimulate hunger or reduce satiety.
- **Slowing metabolism:** Certain medications decrease energy expenditure.
- **Causing fluid retention:** Some drugs lead to bloating and water weight gain.
- **Disrupting insulin sensitivity:** Some medications increase the likelihood of fat storage.

Common Medications That Promote Weight Gain

Antidepressants and Mood Stabilizers

- **Selective serotonin reuptake inhibitors (SSRIs)** (e.g., Prozac, Zoloft): Can increase appetite in some individuals.

- **Tricyclic antidepressants (TCAs) (e.g., amitriptyline):** Are linked to weight gain due to their effects on metabolism.
- **Atypical antipsychotics (e.g., Zyprexa, Seroquel):** One of the most weight-promoting drug classes; increases fat storage and insulin resistance.

Diabetes Medications

- **Insulin:** While essential for diabetes management, promotes fat storage and can cause hypoglycemia, increasing hunger and calorie consumption.
- **Sulfonylureas (e.g., glipizide, glyburide):** Stimulate insulin production but are associated with weight gain.

Blood Pressure Medications

- **Beta-blockers (e.g., metoprolol, propranolol):** Can slow metabolism and reduce energy expenditure.
- **Calcium channel blockers (e.g., amlodipine):** May contribute to fluid retention and bloating.

Steroids for Inflammation and Autoimmune Conditions

- **Corticosteroids (e.g., prednisone):** Known to cause significant weight gain; can increase appetite, fluid retention, and fat redistribution (especially in the abdomen).

ASK YOUR DOCTOR: ARE THERE WEIGHT-NEUTRAL ALTERNATIVES?

If you suspect that your medication may be contributing to weight gain, talk to your doctor. In many cases, there are weight-neutral alternatives available. Some newer antidepressants and diabetes medications, for example, have been shown to be weight neutral or even promote weight loss.

6. Lifestyle Factors

While many of the lifestyle factors discussed here have been touched on throughout this chapter, it's worth wrapping them up in one place to see the full picture. Though obesity is influenced by the many external factors we've addressed already, lifestyle habits still play an important role, especially when it comes to managing weight over time.

Dietary patterns are a major contributor. A high intake of ultraprocessed, calorie-dense, nutrient-poor foods (alongside excess added sugars and saturated fats) can drive weight gain. Irregular meal patterns or eating in response to emotions rather than hunger can also disrupt the body's natural regulatory cues. These patterns are often reinforced by a sedentary lifestyle; long hours sitting at a desk or in front of a screen, paired with low levels of structured or spontaneous movement, make it harder to maintain energy balance.

Sleep and stress further complicate the picture. Getting less than seven hours of sleep at night alters key hunger hormones, increasing ghrelin and decreasing leptin—making people hungrier and more prone to cravings. At the same time, chronic stress can raise one's cortisol level, which encourages fat storage (especially around the abdomen) and often leads to emotional or binge eating. Alcohol can add fuel to this cycle, lowering restraint regarding food, disrupting metabolism, and delivering a boatload of calories with no nutritional value.

Even well-intentioned changes such as quitting smoking have the potential to backfire in the short term. Many people experience temporary weight gain after quitting due to metabolic and appetite changes. All of this unfolds under the umbrella of your broader environment, where access to healthy food, time for self-care, and time and space for exercise aren't evenly distributed.

The constant presence of quick fixes such as fast food and sugary drinks further stacks the odds against you.

In sum, lifestyle factors don't tell the whole story, but they do shape it. They interact with biology and environment in ways that can either ease the path to better health or make it feel like an uphill climb. Seeing them in the larger context as pieces of a complex system is key to moving forward with clarity.

Diagnosing Overweight and Obesity

Now that we've looked at what obesity is and what causes it, let's talk about how we diagnose it. Body mass index (BMI) has long been the standard tool for diagnosing obesity and overweight, but it is an outdated, imprecise measure. Because it measures the ratio between your height and weight, it treats all types of weight the same—whether it is from fat, muscle, or bone. A person with a BMI of 30 or more receives a diagnosis of obesity, and a person with a BMI between 27 and 29.9 is considered to have overweight. However, many people with a "normal" BMI (between 18.5 and 24.9) have high visceral fat and poor metabolic health; this can happen particularly with older adults who have low muscle mass. On the other hand, athletes with high muscle mass end up with a "high" BMI and can be classified as being overweight or having obesity when they're actually in excellent health.

Here's an important nuance that is often overlooked: When people hear that BMI is inaccurate, they often assume that that's because it overdiagnoses obesity. In reality, the opposite is far more common. BMI frequently underdiagnoses obesity, especially in people who appear to be in a "normal" weight range but actually have high levels of visceral fat or very low lean muscle mass. These are patients who can be at a high risk for developing metabolic complications—yet their BMI may not reflect that risk, leaving them undertreated. Many of my patients come in thinking they are simply carrying excess weight and are surprised to learn that they clinically have obesity.

Why do doctors still use BMI to diagnose obesity, even though most of them know that it's an imprecise tool? Well, it's inexpensive, quick, and easy to calculate—and it works for broad population studies, even though it falls short for assessing an individual's health. Despite its flaws, BMI remains the standard for medical records and insurance purposes. Most insurance companies require patients to meet specific BMI thresholds in order to qualify for obesity-related treatments.

But doctors who specialize in obesity medicine rarely rely on BMI alone. Instead, we use body composition analysis, which gives us a much more accurate understanding of an individual's health. **Body composition** refers to the proportion of fat, muscle, bone, and water in your body. Instead of prioritizing weight, it tells you how much of your body is made of fat versus lean mass (such as muscle and organs). Your body composition is determined by an MRI, a DEXA scan or a bioelectric impedance analysis scale (BIA). (I'll explain what these machines are on page 120.)

According to the Obesity Medicine Association:

- **For women,** a body fat percentage of 18 to 28 percent is considered healthy, and anything greater than 32 percent indicates that you have obesity.
- **For men,** a healthy body fat percentage is 10 to 20 percent, and anything greater than 25 percent indicates that you have obesity.

Body fat percentage provides a much clearer picture of your overall health than BMI alone. If you've spent years (or a lifetime) trying to lower your BMI by lowering the number you see on the scale, it can be difficult to deprioritize weight, but once you understand body composition, it becomes clear that these measures are only one part of the picture.

Your body composition is the most crucial measurement you'll track on your GLP-1 journey. I'll be encouraging you to keep an eye on your body composition at home to make sure you're losing fat and not muscle and to confirm that you're making progress at a safe, effective pace. We'll get into all the details of measuring your progress in chapter 5.

> ### Other Metrics for Health and Weight Assessment
>
> Like body fat percentage, the following measurements can provide a more accurate assessment of your body composition and metabolic health than BMI.
>
> - **Visceral fat measurements:** High visceral fat increases risk for heart disease, diabetes, and metabolic disorders. It can be measured using tools such as DEXA scans, MRIs, or BIA devices (which we'll discuss below).
>
> - **Metabolic health markers:** Some key lab tests to measure metabolic health include:
>   - **Fasting glucose and insulin levels:** Assesses insulin resistance.
>   - **Hemoglobin A1c (HbA1c):** Measures long-term blood sugar levels.
>   - **Lipid profile:** Looks at cholesterol and triglyceride levels.
>   - **Inflammatory markers (CRP, IL-6, etc.):** Are elevated in people with metabolic syndrome.
>
> - **Waist-to-hip ratio and waist circumference:** With this simple but effective method of assessing fat distribution, you just need to measure your waist and hips. A high waist circumference is strongly linked to metabolic disease.

Understanding these additional metrics will help you become a better-informed and more empowered patient. If you're working with an obesity specialist, they may look at some of these metrics in addition to body composition. If you're in a more generalized medical setting, knowing which tests and measurements can help paint a clear picture of your overall health might result in more targeted, personalized care, leading to a better long-term outcome.

A New Era for Understanding Obesity

Dear reader, I hope that after this chapter, you no longer see obesity as a simple matter of willpower or personal failure. It is not about how well you follow advice or how much discipline you have. It is a complex, chronic condition shaped by genetics, hormones, trauma, environmental triggers, medications, sleep, and even the food system you were born into. Some of these factors were set into motion long before you were born; others accumulated quietly over time. What's important to know is this: **It's not your fault.** You don't need to "try harder"; you just need to understand your body and finally work with it, not against it.

Obesity is also about a medical community that has long overlooked or misunderstood this disease and, in doing so, has often failed the patients most affected by it. Remember, it is only since 2013 that the AMA has approached obesity as an actual disease, rather than as a motivation problem.

While the history of obesity treatment is full of blind spots and oversights, we are finally entering a new era—one defined by better science, better understanding, and better tools. At the center of this medical evolution are GLP-1 medications, a class of therapies that work with the body's natural systems to help people regulate their appetite, improve their metabolic health, and, yes, finally achieve meaningful and lasting fat loss.

They might sound new, maybe even too good to be true—but they're neither. They're built on decades of research, rooted in hormones your body already makes, and their discovery is one of the most fascinating stories in modern medicine. That's where we'll go next.

CHAPTER 2

Enter GLP-1s: A New Era of Weight Management

You're reading this because GLP-1 medications have sparked your interest—and rightly so. This class of therapy represents one of the most significant advancements in obesity and metabolic care in decades. But if you're feeling hesitant, even a bit skeptical, you're not alone. To many people, GLP-1s seem to have appeared overnight—suddenly everywhere, hailed as the next big thing. It's understandable to have questions when something gains attention so quickly.

But GLP-1 medications are not new; far from it. These medications are the result of more than two decades of research and careful refinement. They were first developed to treat type 2 diabetes, and over time, scientists began to recognize their powerful effects on appetite, weight regulation, and metabolic health.

Understanding where GLP-1 medications come from and how they evolved from an unnamed hormone to a major player in modern medicine can help demystify how they work and strengthen your confidence in using them. This chapter is your behind-the-scenes look at how a molecule produced by your own body became the foundation of one of the most promising treatments in obesity medicine. Let me rewind to where it all began—with a gut hormone that helps regulate blood sugar and appetite in response to food.

A Brief History of GLP-1s

The development of GLP-1 medications is a story marked by scientific curiosity, unexpected discoveries, and bold decisions. It includes setbacks and breakthroughs, unlikely collaborations, and a key figure who trusted his scientific instincts—and changed the course of obesity and metabolic treatment.

In the early 1980s, Dr. Svetlana Mojsov, working with Dr. Joel Habener and their colleagues at Massachusetts General Hospital and Harvard Medical School, discovered that our small intestines naturally produce a hormone that helps the body release insulin when the blood sugar level is high. They named it glucagon-like peptide-1, or GLP-1. It was a major breakthrough in understanding how the body controls blood sugar. Before, we had thought of insulin as the main driver of glucose control, but we didn't know that there was a precursor of insulin that our body produced as we ate our meals.

As promising as that discovery was, developing a pharmaceutical version of GLP-1 posed a major challenge, as the hormone is naturally very short lived. Once it is secreted, an enzyme called DPP-4 breaks it down within two to four minutes. While the discovery was an important educational advancement, scientists couldn't translate the mechanism into an impactful drug due to the hormone's short life. At least not yet.

It wasn't until 1992 that Dr. John Eng, an endocrinologist and researcher at the James J. Peters Department of Veterans Affairs Medical Center in the Bronx, made a discovery that would alter the course of weight loss (and humanity) forever. As a diabetes specialist and researcher, Dr. Eng was interested in finding new hormones in the human body. His scientific curiosity led him down an unexpected path—one that required confronting a molecule once considered more problematic than promising. He wanted to learn more about how to stimulate insulin production in the pancreas, which, in turn, helps regulate blood sugar. Previous discoveries had shown that something in the venom of the Gila monster, one of the few venomous lizards in the world, might be able to stimulate pancreatic activity under certain conditions.

Inspired by those studies, Dr. Eng contacted a serpentarium in Utah for a preserved sample of Gila monster venom. From that sample, he was able to isolate a compound he named exendin-4, which closely resembled GLP-1. The difference? Unlike the short-lived version produced by our bodies, the exendin-4 from the Gila lizard's venom resisted rapid degradation, making it a promising drug candidate. Dr. Eng worked with diabetes patients every day at the VA, and he knew that the discovery could potentially offer a new treatment option.

Despite the breakthrough, Dr. Eng initially struggled to find support. The VA declined to pursue a patent for the discovery, so he and his wife personally paid for it out of pocket. But developing a drug candidate requires extensive research and resources—not to mention hundreds of millions of dollars—and because of that, Dr. Eng knew he would need to partner with a pharmaceutical company for his discovery to go anywhere. For two years, he pitched pharmaceutical companies about exendin-4's potential without success—until he decided to attend the American Diabetes Association annual meeting in 1996 and present his findings. In a conference hall crowded with other presenters, he stood next to a simple poster that outlined his research, and he explained his findings on exendin-4 to anyone who would listen.

By chance, Andrew Young, the head of physiology at the small biotech firm Amylin Pharmaceuticals, walked by and took notice. Amylin had been working on GLP-1-related therapies but kept running against the hormone's short lifespan in the body. Young quickly realized that Dr. Eng might have found the solution they'd been looking for. As he took in Dr. Eng's poster, a representative from the much larger Eli Lilly and Company slowed to a stop and began reading over Eng's shoulder. Suddenly Eng's presentation would cause a race to see who could secure his work.

The smaller and more agile Amylin ultimately won out, and over time, researchers found a way to synthesize the compound exendin-4 as exenatide, sold under the brand name Byetta. In 2005, Byetta became the first GLP-1-based drug approved by the FDA. It offered a brand-new approach to the treatment of type 2 diabetes, enabling people to regulate their blood sugar through a different mechanism. Eventually Lilly came back and partnered with Amylin, investing a whopping $325 million to keep the drug research going.

Dr. Eng's steadfast belief in his discovery laid the foundation of a revolution in diabetes and obesity treatment. The story is a testament to curiosity, determination, self-conviction, and the power of coming together for the common good.

So was the collaboration happily ever after? Not quite. Byetta was the first GLP-1 medication used as a treatment for type 2 diabetes, but there were some kinks to work out before it evolved into the GLP-1s we know and love today. Byetta users needed to inject the medication twice a day, thirty minutes before breakfast and thirty minutes before dinner. That timing was impractical and easy to forget; many people would begin to eat before their injection or accidentally miss their second dose. It also had unpleasant side effects, such as pronounced nausea and vomiting. Some people felt so nauseous that they felt the need to throw up shortly after their injections. Needless to say, compliance was low, and the drug didn't make waves. An effective drug no one wants to take isn't an effective drug.

In 2010, Novo Nordisk introduced an improved version of GLP-1 therapy with the development of liraglutide. Sold under the brand name Victoza, the medication needed to be injected only once a day, which was a major improvement from Byetta's twice-daily regimen. With its fewer side effects and greater convenience, Victoza showed better patient compliance and gained traction quickly.

Around the same time, researchers were also working to develop a version of exenatide that was even longer acting. In 2012, the FDA approved Bydureon (exenatide extended-release). It was the first GLP-1 medication that could be taken just once a week. That was a significant step forward, providing people with type 2 diabetes a more convenient option for managing their blood sugar with fewer daily disruptions. Still, Bydureon also had its drawbacks. Its extended-release formulation used a mechanism that caused some patients to develop lumps at the injection site—definitely an unpleasant (and sometimes even painful) side effect. The foundation was strong, but there was room for improvement.

Meanwhile, Victoza was gaining more widespread, consistent usage, and we endocrinologists began to notice a surprising side effect: weight loss. (Remember, at that point, the drugs were indicated and approved only for treating type 2 diabetes.) It wasn't until medications such as liraglutide were used in real-world clinical settings that we were able to see the way they influence the brain's reward system, helping patients lose significant amounts of weight safely and sustainably. Soon enough, we began using Victoza "off label" for weight loss—especially when we saw how well our patients without diabetes responded to it. Because liraglutide stimulates insulin production only when blood sugar is elevated, patients with normal glucose levels could lose weight without experiencing hypoglycemia (low blood sugar), which is a common side effect of many diabetes drugs.

Encouraged by those results, Novo Nordisk formally studied liraglutide as a treatment for obesity. In 2014, it launched Saxenda, the first GLP-1 medication approved by the FDA for chronic weight management, independent of a type 2 diabetes diagnosis.

Though liraglutide needed to be administered with only a once-daily injection, some patients still felt that it was an "extreme" length to go to for weight loss—or even glucose control. They asked, "If I don't need insulin, then why do I still have to inject myself daily?" Fair question.

But remember, earlier efforts to simplify dosing (such as Bydureon) hadn't quite hit the mark for ease or comfort. So back to the lab the researchers went—this time to make a drug that not only worked physiologically but fit into the rhythms of everyday life comfortably, with fewer side effects. The result? Semaglutide (brand names: Ozempic and Wegovy), which required an injection only once a week.

Yes, Ozempic became the poster child of GLP-1s. Unless you've been living under a rock, you've caught wind of the name or at least heard the catchy marketing song. It created a cultural moment. It became a Hollywood accessory. It even, arguably, spawned a new type of face.

There are now even more players in the game. Tirzepatide by Eli Lilly (brand names Zepbound and Mounjaro) came onto the scene in 2022. Tirzepatide is a little different from everything we've talked about so far. Up until now, all the medications in this class worked by mimicking just one hormone: GLP-1. However, tirzepatide is the first dual drug of its class: It mimics both GLP-1 and glucagon-inhibiting protein, or GIP.

GLP-1 and GIP are both incretins, a group of naturally occurring gut hormones that help regulate blood sugar, insulin secretion, digestion, and appetite. These hormones appear to work better as a team and help people lose more weight, often with fewer side effects, compared to older GLP-1-only medications. By offering a new level of effectiveness, tirzepatide is changing what we thought was possible in obesity and diabetes care.

But wait—there's more! Eli Lilly is already working on the next evolution in this class of medications—a *triple* incretin called retatrutide, which is currently in Phase 3 clinical trials. Retatrutide adds one more hormone to the mix: glucagon. Together, these three hormones work to regulate appetite, blood sugar, fat metabolism, and energy expenditure, which could lead to even greater weight loss and metabolic improvements than current medications do. While it's not yet FDA approved, retatrutide is showing serious promise, and hopefully it will be available by the time you read this.

And that's not the only new drug in the pipeline. Several others are currently in late-stage clinical trials. Their mechanisms differ slightly. Some build on GLP-1s by adding another hormone the same way that retatrutide does; others target entirely new pathways involved in appetite, fat storage, and metabolism. Most of these are expected to roll out over the next few years, pending FDA approval:

- **Orforglipron (Eli Lilly):** A once-daily oral GLP-1 receptor agonist, expected as early as 2026
- **CagriSema (Novo Nordisk):** A powerful injectable combo of semaglutide (GLP-1) and an amylin analog, likely available by 2026
- **Survodutide (Boehringer Ingelheim):** A dual-acting injectable that targets GLP-1 and glucagon receptors, projected for 2027 or later

- **MariTide (Amgen):** An experimental GLP-1 agonist and a once-a-month injection that also blocks GIP signaling, likely available in 2028 or beyond
- **Bimagrumab (Eli Lilly):** A myostatin inhibitor aimed at reducing fat and preserving muscle; possible release in or after 2028
- **Monlunabant (Novo Nordisk):** A CB1 receptor blocker that targets appetite via the brain's reward system; still in early trials, with potential availability after 2028

Oral GLP-1s

In 2019, the FDA approved the first oral GLP-1 medication for the treatment of type 2 diabetes: Rybelsus, a daily pill version of semaglutide. There were high expectations for an oral alternative to injections, but despite the convenience, they haven't gained the same traction as their injectable counterparts—and for good reason. Oral semaglutide must be absorbed through the stomach, which limits the amount of the drug that reaches the bloodstream. To match the metabolic effects of injectable GLP-1s such as Ozempic or Wegovy, much higher doses would be needed, but higher doses are often poorly tolerated. Oral semaglutide has been associated with more gastrointestinal side effects than its injectable counterpart.

Glucose control with oral semaglutide is comparable to that of the injectable form, but its impact on weight loss is significantly weaker. The combination of lower tolerable dosing, inconsistent absorption, and higher rates of GI side effects has made it less effective as an anti-obesity treatment.

At the time of this writing, no oral GLP-1 has been FDA approved for weight loss. Research and development are ongoing, but the injectable versions remain the standard of care for both metabolic disease and obesity treatment.

A Timeline of GLP-1 Development Milestones

1980s: Discovery of GLP-1
Biochemist Dr. Svetlana Mojsov identified the GLP-1 molecule for the first time. She also theorized that GLP-1 was an incretin. Later, in collaboration with Dr. Joel Habener and colleagues, the function of GLP-1 was identified.

1992: Discovery of Exendin-4
Dr. John Eng discovers exendin-4, a GLP-1-like compound in Gila monster venom. Exendin-4 is longer-lasting than human GLP-1 and ideal for drug development.

2005: FDA Approval of Byetta (Exenatide)
Byetta is the first GLP-1 receptor agonist approved in the US to treat type 2 diabetes and was developed from exendin-4. It's approved for type 2 diabetes and requires twice-daily injections.

2010: FDA Approval of Victoza (Liraglutide)
Victoza is a GLP-1 approved in the US to treat type 2 diabetes, with improved tolerability and ease of use; it requires once-daily injections.

2012: FDA Approval of Bydureon (Exenatide Extended-Release)
The first once-weekly GLP-1 injection, Byudereon provides longer-acting control for type 2 diabetes.

2014: FDA Approval of Saxenda (Liraglutide 3.0 milligrams)
The first GLP-1 to be FDA approved for chronic weight management (not just diabetes) in adults living with obesity or overweight, plus a related condition.

2017: FDA Approval of Ozempic (Semaglutide)
A once-weekly GLP-1 receptor agonist for type 2 diabetes, Ozempic shows stronger effects on blood sugar and weight loss.

2019: FDA Approval of Rybelsus (Semaglutide)
The first daily oral GLP-1 approved for the treatment of type 2 diabetes.

2021: FDA Approval of Wegovy (Semaglutide 2.4 milligrams)
Wegovy is a higher-dose semaglutide, becoming the first once-weekly GLP-1 approved specifically for chronic weight management in adults without diabetes.

2022: FDA Approval of Mounjaro (Tirzepatide)
Mounjaro is the first dual incretin (GLP-1 + GIP) therapy approved for type 2 diabetes. It has improved weight loss results, even compared to semaglutide.

2023: FDA Approval of Zepbound (Tirzepatide)
Tirzepatide receives a second FDA approval, this time for chronic weight management under the brand name Zepbound.

Ongoing: Retatrutide in Development (Triple Incretin)
This triple incretin therapy (GLP-1 + GIP + glucagon) is in clinical trials and shows potential for unprecedented weight loss and improved metabolic health.

How Do GLP-1s Work in the Body?

As I've already touched on, GLP-1 is a hormone that your body makes and releases naturally in your gut after you eat. But our body's natural GLP-1 breaks down quickly and doesn't cross the blood-brain barrier in meaningful amounts. That's where pharmaceutical GLP-1s come in.

The medications I talked about above are what we call GLP-1 receptor agonists. They are synthetic versions of the natural GLP-1 hormone or, in some cases, slightly altered versions that act in the same way but last longer in the body. We call them receptor agonists because they mimic our natural GLP-1 and activate the same receptor. Many people and publications refer to GLP-1 receptor agonists as GLP-1s for short.

These synthetic, long-acting versions have a longer impact on our brain's reward system and the way our body perceives satiety than our naturally produced GLP-1 does. But how exactly do they cause weight loss? The primary mechanism is through a sustained caloric deficit. In simple terms, when we consistently take in more calories than we use, the excess is stored as fat tissue in the body. This fat acts as a backup energy reserve for times of scarcity or increased energy demand. But when we take in fewer calories than our body needs, it turns to our fat reserves, breaking down stored fat to use for fuel; this process is called fat oxidation. In other words, to lose fat, we need to consume fewer calories than we burn. But that's not always as easy as it sounds. GLP-1 medications help us create that calorie deficit in three ways:

1. **First, they slow gastric emptying.** This delays food leaving the stomach, leading to greater satiety and reduced appetite.

2. **Second, they enhance the body's satiety signaling.** This happens in part by influencing hormones such as peptide YY and reducing the levels of hunger hormones such as ghrelin,

making your body chemically shift into a state where food just isn't as appealing or urgent as it used to be.

3. **Third—and this is the most interesting part**—they interact with the GLP-1 receptors in the brain, including an area called the amygdala. You're probably already familiar with the amygdala. It's a major processing center for emotions, motivation, and decision-making. No surprise, it's also responsible for emotional and reward-based eating. GLP-1 medications can reduce the dopamine-driven "food noise" that pushes people to snack when they're not hungry or overeat highly palatable foods. (When you're snacking on something so addictive that you idly wonder if it's laced with drugs, blame your amygdala.) By reducing food noise, you don't just feel full sooner; you're actually clearing up the overactive wiring in your brain. Many people describe it as a kind of "mental quieting" regarding food.

The End of Dieting

One of the most revolutionary things about GLP-1 medications is that they make weight loss feel more natural. For many people, that means no more crash diets, no more white knuckling through hunger, and no more obsessing over every bite. That's because they don't just reduce appetite; they recalibrate the entire system that used to drive overeating in the first place.

Instead of having to rely on willpower to resist cravings, you may find that the cravings are gone. You may feel full faster, be satisfied with less food, and genuinely prefer healthier options without forcing yourself to do so.

Think of it this way: Traditional diets teach you to fight your body into changing, while GLP-1 medications create the conditions that make change easier.

What Makes Tirzepatide Different?

While GLP-1 medications such as semaglutide (Ozempic and Wegovy) work by producing the same effects as natural GLP-1 in a more efficient way, tirzepatide, a newer, more powerful medication, is in a class of its own.

As I mentioned earlier, tirzepatide mimics two hormones: GLP-1 and GIP. Like GLP-1, GIP plays a role in managing blood sugar and metabolism. It may also have its own effects on fat storage and energy balance, and when it is combined with GLP-1, the two hormones seem to work synergistically, boosting each other's effects.

What does this dual-action approach mean for you?

Tirzepatide works on both GLP-1 and GIP receptors, creating a broader metabolic effect than GLP-1 alone. This means greater weight loss, better blood sugar control, and, for some people, fewer gastrointestinal side effects. If semaglutide was the breakthrough—like the first iPhone that redefined the landscape—tirzepatide is the next-generation model, building on that innovation with more power and versatility. It builds on the same foundational mechanism as earlier GLP-1 therapies but delivers enhanced performance and broader metabolic benefits. And now retatrutide—next-generation therapy that's already capturing attention across the field—is on the horizon.

While tirzepatide offers significant advantages and may be the starting point for many (if not most) patients, it's not a one-size-fits-all solution. In the next chapter, we'll explore how to choose the GLP-1 medication that best aligns with your health profile, treatment goals, and access to care.

If GLP-1 Medications Aren't New, Why All the Attention Now?

As I mentioned at the beginning of this chapter, the FDA approved the first GLP-1 medication (Byetta) in 2005. So this class of drugs is not new. Before Ozempic, the medical community had seventeen years of experience with them. If these treatments have been around for a long time, why does it seem like they exploded onto the market? There are a couple of factors that have contributed to the current awareness of GLP-1 medications. I've touched on most of them already, but let's bring them all together.

- **The covid-19 pandemic:** Obesity had long been considered a health condition that resulted from a lack of willpower, not a true disease. Covid exposed that obesity can be an acute, high-risk disease—not just a slow, silent health issue. Covid patients with obesity were more likely to experience severe symptoms, had more intensive care unit stays during the pandemic than other groups did, and had higher mortality rates due to infections. For patients with obesity, suddenly their weight wasn't a cosmetic issue that *might* lead to health consequences in the future; it was a real medical risk factor, and they were seeing the consequences *now*. Patients got the message that they didn't have to wait decades to develop a complication from having excess fat. During the pandemic, I had patients with obesity who told me, "I don't want to die from covid. Please help me lose weight." Knowing that they had the tools to help patients meet their goals, the pharmaceutical companies got to work bringing these medications to market, and doctors started prescribing them.
- **Improvements in formulations:** These drugs went from requiring twice-daily injections to once-daily injections to once-weekly injections. The development of a longer-acting medication made them much easier to use and led

to the high rates of medication compliance that we see today. Additionally, the side effects of newer formulations are less severe.

- **FDA approval for weight loss:** Early versions of these medications were approved only for diabetes management. While some physicians had been prescribing them off-label for weight loss for years, the FDA officially approved semaglutide as a treatment for obesity only in 2021.

ACTIVE INGREDIENT	APPROVED FOR DIABETES	APPROVED FOR WEIGHT LOSS
Semaglutide	Ozempic	Wegovy
Tirzepatide	Mounjaro	Zepbound
Liraglutide	Victoza	Saxenda

Understanding FDA Approval and Compounded Meds

If you're considering GLP-1 therapy, there's one key distinction that can significantly affect your treatment experience and safety: whether you're receiving an FDA-approved medication or a compounded version. As of May 22, 2025, compounding pharmacies are no longer legally permitted to compound semaglutide. This change reflects the drug's removal from the FDA's shortage list, which had previously allowed temporary exceptions. Going forward, any semaglutide you receive must come in the form of an FDA-approved product such as Ozempic or Wegovy, or it may not be legally dispensed.

What does that mean in practice? Did compounded semaglutide vanish overnight? Not exactly. Some clinics are attempting to sidestep regulations by altering the drug's formulation or labeling it under slightly different names (calling it a "research peptide," for instance, or combining it with additives to create a *technically different* compound). But this is a gray area of the market and is legally and medically questionable.

Let's break down why the distinction between compounded GLP-1s and FDA-approved drugs matters.

FDA-approved GLP-1 medications—such as Ozempic, Wegovy, Mounjaro, and Zepbound—have gone through years of rigorous clinical trials, safety reviews, and ongoing manufacturing oversight. They are prescription drugs backed by peer-reviewed data and regulatory standards. When you pick one up from your pharmacy, you're getting a product that's been thoroughly vetted for efficacy, consistency, and safety.

Compounded GLP-1 medications, on the other hand, are made by pharmacies that mix or alter ingredients to create custom versions of the drugs. In rare cases, compounded medications exist because they can be lifesavers for special populations, providing workarounds for people who have allergies to certain fillers, need a pediatric dose, or require a medication that's no longer commercially available. But in the case of GLP-1s, the use of custom workarounds has exploded far beyond these typical situations.

Compounded GLP-1 medications became widely normalized during the shortages of 2022 and 2023, providing access to them when FDA-approved options were hard to find. But now that the shortage is over, some patients are still turning to compounded options—sometimes without realizing what they're getting.

Some compounded GLP-1s are sold online or dispensed by med spas—often by practitioners who specialize in aesthetic treatments, not endocrinology or obesity medicine. A licensed healthcare provider does technically need to prescribe the medication, but that doesn't always mean the prescriber is knowledgeable about best practices or monitoring. You can walk into some clinics and walk out with a week's worth of injections without knowing what to do if something goes wrong.

> ### The FDA Approval Process
>
> To better understand how compounded GLP-1s are different from brand-name medications, it helps to know what FDA approval actually entails. Here's what a medication such as semaglutide or tirzepatide goes through before you ever see it on a pharmacy shelf.
>
> - **Preclinical testing:** In vitro (lab) and animal studies are conducted to assess basic safety and biological activity.
> - **Phase 1 trials:** Small studies in healthy volunteers are done to examine safety and dosage.
> - **Phase 2 trials:** Studies in larger groups of people are used to evaluate effectiveness and side effects.
> - **Phase 3 trials:** Large-scale studies in multiple populations confirm the drug's safety and efficacy.
> - **FDA review and inspection:** The FDA conducts a full evaluation of all trial data, labeling, and manufacturing facilities.
> - **Postmarket monitoring:** There is ongoing surveillance of side effects, recalls, and new research data.
>
> Each step takes years and costs millions of dollars. These requirements are in place for a reason: to make sure the drugs you take are consistent, effective, and safe.

If you have access to an FDA-approved GLP-1, that's always the preferred route. These medications have been carefully researched, controlled, and proven to be both safe and effective. But if your only access is through a compounded version—because of cost, insurance, or availability—I would rather you pursue that route safely than go without treatment altogether. The potential of GLP-1s to transform lives is too great to ignore. You will learn how to be an informed consumer in "Using Compounded GLP-1s Safely" in chapter 4.

All About GLP-1 Therapy: FAQ

I'm sure you have lots of questions. For now I'll just address the ones that are about GLP-1 medications themselves. If you're wondering about the more practical and personal aspects of the GLP-1 journey, don't worry, we'll get to all of that; this is just the beginning.

Q: I'm worried that GLP-1s haven't been studied long enough. Am I a guinea pig?

A: Now that you know the history of GLP-1 development, I hope that it's become clearer that GLP-1s aren't as new as they seem. We've been prescribing these drugs successfully for decades, and they're becoming better and better over time. You're not a test subject; you're someone who is taking advantage of a therapy that has already helped many people improve their health and quality of life.

Q: Do I need to worry about side effects?

A: Like any other medication, GLP-1 medications come with potential side effects, but there's a key distinction you should be aware of. Most are secondary effects that typically happen only when the drug isn't used properly or are the same side effects that can occur with any significant weight loss. Later in this book, I'll explain this nuance and how you can use GLP-1 medications in a way that minimizes or avoids the secondary effects related to the medication entirely. For now, here's a quick rundown of the mild side effects that may happen as a direct result of the mechanisms of the medication.

- **Nausea/digestive changes:** Many people experience some degree of nausea when starting a GLP-1 medication because the medication slows the rate at which your stomach empties and sends satiety signals to your brain. It can take a little time for your body to adjust to these changes. You might also experience bloating, constipation, or mild diarrhea, but these digestive changes are usually short-lived and manageable.
- **Headache/fatigue:** Some people report low-level headaches or dips in energy during the adjustment phase. These tend to resolve as your body adapts, especially if you stay on top of your nutrition and hydration.
- **Heartburn/acid reflux:** This can happen due to the slow gastric emptying effect of the drug. The longer food sits in the stomach, the longer the digestive acid remains. This can increase the symptoms of acid reflux. It is important to have small meals during treatment.
- **Dehydration:** This isn't a direct effect of the medication, but it is something that many GLP-1 users report. Normally we consume liquids along with meals, but if you are having small meals, you will be drinking less fluids. Proactively drink liquids throughout the day.

Q: How are GLP-1 receptor agonists different from weight loss drugs of the past?

A: Traditional weight loss drugs artificially suppress appetite by using central nervous system stimulants. They were designed to override your body's signals and came with some serious side effects that made their long-term use dangerous. Instead of forcing short-term appetite suppression, GLP-1 medications mimic a naturally produced hormone and help correct underlying hormonal imbalances. They are also safe for long-term and maintenance use (more on this in chapter 7).

Other FDA-Approved Weight Loss Medications

The FDA has approved several medications for chronic weight management in adults with obesity or weight-related health conditions. Each of these works a little differently: some suppress appetite, some reduce fat absorption, some target cravings. This book focuses on GLP-1 receptor agonists, but it's helpful to understand the broader landscape. The chart below gives a quick overview of each approved drug and how it works.

MEDICATION	MECHANISM
Orlistat (Xenical, Alli)	Blocks the absorption of some fat from the food you eat.
Phentermine	Suppresses appetite by stimulating the central nervous system; short-term use only.
Phentermine/ topiramate (Qysmia)	Suppresses appetite and increases feelings of fullness.
Naltrexone/ buproprion (Contrave)	Targets areas of the brain involved in reward and hunger; reduces cravings and appetite.

GLP-1 receptor agonist (semaglutide, tirzepatide, liraglutide)	Mimics hormones naturally released in the gut. Slows gastric emptying, increases satiety, reduces appetite, and regulates blood sugar. Also blunts reward-based eating.
Setmelanotide (Imcivree)	Limited to people who have been diagnosed with rare genetic disorders that affect the MC4R pathway. Restores proper signaling in the brain to regulate hunger and energy balance, promoting weight loss.

Q: How quickly will I lose weight?

A: This is a great question with a slightly complicated answer that we will explore more deeply in chapter 5. Here's the short version: This journey is not a sprint; it's more of a long-distance run. Depending on factors such as the medication, the dosage, and your genetics, starting weight, and age, the pace of weight loss will vary. Some weeks you may lose more, some weeks less, and some weeks not at all. And that can be normal. The goal here isn't rapid weight loss; it's sustainable progress that will protect your muscles, support your metabolism, and help you feel your best—long term.

Q: Can I improve my body's GLP-1 production via GLP-1 "booster" or "activator" supplements, gummies, or drink mixes?

A: No, and any product that markets itself this way should raise red flags. Sure, there are things that may help stimulate your body's natural GLP-1 production, but remember what you just learned: Our body's natural GLP-1 doesn't last for more than a few minutes and doesn't cross the blood-brain barrier in significant amounts. Because the supplements on the market, such as the ones made with berberine, don't address these factors, they won't have any significant impact on weight loss.

Q: Do I have to stay on the medications for the rest of my life? Are they safe to stay on forever?

A: The first question is a little nuanced, and we'll be getting into it in greater detail in the next chapter. For now, I can tell you that GLP-1s are designed for long-term use—remember, we're treating a chronic medical condition, not a willpower problem—and they are safe to stay on for the long term. Still, my goal is always to keep you at the smallest possible dose, and some patients do have success with intermittent use or can eventually wean off them entirely.

Q. I've heard a lot of conflicting information about the benefits and risks of GLP-1s. How do I know who and what to trust?

A: In our current media landscape, it's all too easy for sensational headlines to drown out science. The truth is often distorted or oversimplified for sound bites, and there are even people on social media who make things up to fearmonger and gain views and clicks. Even well-meaning friends or family members may form opinions based on incomplete or misleading stories. When evaluating claims, always check the source. Listen only to information backed by peer-reviewed research or published by trusted medical organizations. That's exactly why I poured so much effort into writing this book: to provide a clear, credible guide when others—even some healthcare providers—may still be catching up. Let this guide be your experienced companion to cut through the noise.

Q: So what's the catch?

A: Ah, the hidden twist—the unspoken message saying, "You'll still have to suffer for years to earn your health." Let me be clear: You can set that idea aside. The belief that effective treatment must come with punishment or sacrifice is rooted in stigma, not science. We've been conditioned to think of weight gain as something we did wrong, and therefore, losing weight has to feel like punishment, right? It can feel disorienting—even suspicious—to hear that a medication can have so many benefits without some kind of hidden downside or ominous trade-off. But the truth is, these are safe, evidence-based treatments that are generally well tolerated, and they address the root causes of appetite dysregulation and weight gain. That said, GLP-1 therapy isn't something you can do on autopilot. You still have to show up, especially when it comes to nutrition, movement, and mindset—but now you'll have support that actually works.

Q: Are there any benefits beyond weight loss?

A: GLP-1 therapy is showing some promising benefits beyond diabetes management and weight loss to impact multiple systems throughout the body. As with the medication's side effects, some of the benefits are the direct results of the synthetic GLP-1 hormone, while others are secondary benefits that occur as a result of weight loss and the accompanying improved metabolic health.

- **GLP-1 agonists may help improve obstructive sleep apnea (OSA).** Sleep apnea is commonly linked with excess weight, and weight loss from GLP-1s can reduce airway obstruction by reducing fat around the neck and upper airway. Emerging research suggests that GLP-1s may also have direct neurological or inflammatory effects that influence airway control independent of weight loss.

- **GLP-1 agonists reduce the risk of heart attack and stroke.** Large-scale studies have shown that GLP-1s can reduce the risk of major cardiovascular events, even in patients who don't experience dramatic weight loss. This may be due to their effects on blood vessel function, inflammation, and cholesterol metabolism.
- **GPL-1 agonists may improve brain health.** Most exciting (in my opinion) is the growing research into the potential neurological benefits of these drugs. As we learned earlier, we have receptors for GLP-1s in our brains, and preclinical studies are showing that GLP-1 analogs may reduce inflammation, oxidative stress, and amyloid plaque buildup in the brain, which are all factors implicated in Alzheimer's disease and other forms of dementia. Clinical trials are currently under way to determine their ability to prevent or slow down cognitive decline.
- **GLP-1 agonists are also being studied for their potential to treat addiction,** including nicotine, alcohol, and even opioid addiction. By acting on dopamine-driven reward pathways in the brain, GLP-1s may help dampen the compulsive drive that fuels addictive behaviors.
- **GLP-1 agonists can indirectly slow down the progression of certain cancers.** GLP-1s are *not* a treatment for cancer. But we know that visceral fat promotes inflammation, which can, in turn, weaken the immune system. By reducing inflammation, your immune system is free to work during your cancer treatment.

LAUREN'S STORY

My entire life, I had been a dancer, and I've modeled since the age of thirteen. Nutrition was ingrained in my lifestyle. But the pressures of those early years led to exercise obsession and disordered eating when I was a teen. With a family history of diabetes and lupus and an early diagnosis of hypothyroidism at sixteen, I became hypervigilant.

I had worked incredibly hard to find peace and love my body. I trained it, dressed it joyfully, and felt for the most part that I was blessed to have it.

Then a series of hardships changed everything: a cab accident, multiple miscarriages, and two major surgeries to remove fibroids. Later, I had more surgeries to remove tumors from my spine, bladder, and rectum.

In the middle of the pandemic—exhausted, in tears, and in pain—I was living in a body I no longer recognized. My organs were taxed. I wasn't eating. My apartment had become a home gym, strewn with equipment in a desperate attempt to regain some control.

My appointment for a GLP-1 changed my life, quite honestly. It gave me my life back. Managing my thyroid, my prediabetes, and hormones finally felt possible. GLP-1 therapy has allowed me to come back to myself—as an athlete, as a performer, as a woman. I am beyond grateful.

The Promise of GLP-1 Therapy

Throughout this chapter, I've laid the foundation for understanding how GLP-1s work and why they matter. Up until now, thinking of obesity as a medical condition may have felt a lot like giving up. It can be discouraging to be told that something that impacts your health is out of your control, especially when you're not offered a clear path forward. But now that we have a treatment that directly addresses the biological drivers of obesity, understanding it as a medical condition no longer means that you are powerless.

That's also what makes this moment so, *so* exciting and empowering. **Obesity is not a choice; choosing to treat it is.** And choosing GLP-1 treatment is not a shortcut or a cheat code; it's a way to reclaim your health with the very best tools science has to offer.

This is not just a breakthrough for individuals; it's a paradigm shift for medicine and for the way society views weight and health. Can you see why I'm so passionate about GLP-1 therapy? I hope you are, too.

CHAPTER 3

Are GLP-1s Right for You?: Evaluating Your Candidacy and Risks

We've now established that excess weight isn't a willpower problem; it's a result of a chronic, multifactorial medical condition and other factors beyond our control. And we've explored the emergence of GLP-1 medications, which are the most comprehensive and effective treatments we've ever had for addressing this condition.

Given the scale of that breakthrough, it's only natural to wonder: What does this mean for me? Could something this big—this transformative—actually change *my* life?

For most people reading this book, and maybe you, weight has been a central struggle for years, even decades or a lifetime. It may have consumed your energy, emotional bandwidth, and self-worth for so long that it can be hard to imagine what life might feel like on the other side. But I can tell you this: You don't have to live with this constant internal battle anymore. That other side is within reach—and most likely, GLP-1s can help you get there.

What's Your Weight Story?
When a patient comes to me asking if they may be a candidate for GLP-1s, the first thing I do is have them tell me their story. For new patients, we spend nearly the whole hour of their first appointment talking about their history with their weight.

I ask them, "At what age did you first become conscious of your weight?" For many of my patients, that awareness didn't start during adulthood or even adolescence but in childhood. But not every story looks the same. Perhaps they didn't struggle with their weight while growing up, but something shifted later in life—menopause, a pregnancy, a new medication, or an injury—that made their weight harder to manage. Maybe they follow the healthy eating guidelines that their doctor recommended, but no matter how hard they try to lose the extra pounds, their body doesn't seem to respond. Maybe they *have* managed to keep their weight under control for periods of time, but maintaining that weight felt like a full-time job; it required constant vigilance about nutrition and exercise, and small slipups put them right back to where they'd started.

Over the years, I've heard from countless patients. Each one's experience with weight was shaped by different circumstances, struggles, and milestones. I see patients who have lost hope, who have made losing weight their lifetime mission without an end. And while no two people's experiences are alike, I've noticed certain patterns that tend to come up again and again. Here, I'll walk through a few of the most common weight stories that I encounter in my practice. These categories aren't meant to put anyone in a box but to help you recognize the most common ways that weight struggles can shape our lives. Please know that these categories aren't exhaustive, and elements of one weight story might overlap with another. Weight journeys are both dynamic and multifaceted.

My goal with sharing these weight stories is to provide a starting broad framework to help you understand the challenges GLP-1s can help address. If any of these weight stories resonate with you, there's a good chance that you could benefit from a GLP-1—and not just as your last option. In fact, it should be your *first* option. Why suffer through decades of diets and spend all your time, money, and willpower to "earn" the right to seek medical treatment for a medical problem? If your weight feels like a constant source of distress, limitation, or frustration, or if you've found it impossible to maintain progress despite your best efforts, that's enough to start a conversation. I give you permission to take GLP-1 therapy seriously as a valid and proactive first step.

The Lifelong Struggle

Patients with this type of story have been battling their weight since childhood or adolescence. Often they've been on diets and may have already felt that their body was a problem that needed to be fixed, as early as age eight years old. Some were sent to "weight loss camps," enrolled in extreme exercise programs, or placed on restrictive food plans before they even understood what calories were. Others may have watched their mother diet, restrict her eating, and speak negatively about her own body, projecting her body image problems onto them in the process.

This early conditioning hits hard and runs *deep*. It shapes how we relate to food, to exercise, to self-image, and to self-worth, and it can persist for decades. By the time these patients reach their twenties, thirties, or forties, they've tried everything, yet still find themselves trapped in a cycle of losing and regaining weight. For many, the struggle has taken up two-thirds of their life. This group often carries emotional scars from being blamed for something that was never fully in their control. Some patients tell me that food takes up permanent real estate in their minds. Thoughts about food are a low-level hum that never shuts off, and they feel that they're fighting a war with these thoughts twenty-four hours a day, seven days a week.

The Sudden Shift

If you are like some of my patients, your weight may have been difficult but manageable—until it wasn't. Perhaps you grew up athletic and active, used to carefully watch what you ate, and got regular exercise. For years, everything was fine, but once you decreased your level of activity—maybe in college or young adulthood—the weight crept on quickly. Or even though you continued that active lifestyle, something suddenly shifted. Perimenopause, midlife hormonal changes, or just the natural aging process changed your physiology, and suddenly your habits stopped working. You're doing even more than before—eating whole foods, working out, tracking macros—but the weight won't budge. Your body is no longer responding the way it used to, and it feels as though you're fighting an uphill battle against your biology.

The Life Event That Changes Everything

Patients with this weight story often haven't struggled with their weight historically, but they experienced a major event that led to significant weight gain: trauma, pregnancy, injury, surgery, or a stressful period. Because of time, hormones, or other responsibilities, these patients usually come in saying, "This isn't my normal—I just haven't been able to get back to my baseline."

GLP-1 Eligibility

I've shared the three types of weight stories on pages 56 to 57 because they reflect real lives, not just numbers on the scale. Your lived experience often reveals more about your needs than a number on a chart does. Unfortunately, though, the reality is that insurance companies and prescribing guidelines still rely on specific clinical criteria. GLP-1 medications are currently FDA approved to treat two primary categories of patients:

1. Those with type 2 diabetes.

2. Those who have obesity or overweight (as defined by their BMI) and at least one weight-related comorbidity. A comorbidity is any current medical complication caused by or related to having excess weight. Common comorbidities include, but are not limited to, sleep apnea, osteoarthritis, prediabetes, and hypertension.

The FDA provides additional guidelines based on BMI to help you determine if you are in the second category:

- A BMI of 30 or above qualifies you as a candidate for GLP-1 treatment.
- A BMI of 27 or above also qualifies—if you also have a comorbidity.

Clinical eligibility is one thing. Being able to get the medication is another. While we now understand that BMI is a deeply flawed and outdated measure for the reasons I discussed in chapter 2, it remains the standard diagnostic tool in most clinical settings. The BMI-based diagnostic guidelines above are what insurance companies use to determine coverage for your medication. Many insurance companies have also added their own hoops to jump through and often require even stricter criteria than the FDA does. In reality, many insurers are doing everything they can *not* to cover these medications. Some require a BMI of 40 or above, effectively limiting coverage to the most extreme cases. Others may cover only a certain brand; for example, if an insurance company has made a deal with Novo Nordisk, it will cover only Ozempic or Wegovy.

We'll talk more about insurance and cost in the next chapter, but here's the bottom line: If you don't meet the textbook definitions of having obesity, overweight, or diabetes, or even if you have a "normal" BMI, that should *not* disqualify you from discussing GLP-1s with your doctor. These medications have been life-changing for many patients whose struggles were never fully captured by BMI or traditional diagnostic criteria.

GLP-1S AND SMALLER WEIGHT LOSS GOALS

You might be wondering whether you can take a GLP-1 medication if you want to lose only ten to fifteen pounds. The answer is yes if these two scenarios apply to you:

- Your body composition reveals that you have more fat to lose than you realized.
- Weight management is taking over your life; it feels like a full-time job, and you've already been following lifestyle recommendations and healthy habits without seeing results.

GLP-1s and Preexisting Conditions

Many patients assume that their preexisting medical conditions automatically disqualify them from using GLP-1 medications—but that's not always the case. In fact, GLP-1s can be safely used by people who have common health conditions. Some scenarios may require closer monitoring or a personalized approach by your doctor, but most conditions are not outright contraindications that make a GLP-1 medication out of the question. Below, you'll find a chart that groups preexisting conditions into three categories:

- **Not a contraindication:** GLP-1s are generally safe in these scenarios.
- **Speak to an experienced provider:** Case-by-case consideration is needed.
- **True contraindication:** GLP-1s should not be used if you or a first-degree family member has this.

NOT A CONTRAINDICATION	SPEAK TO AN EXPERIENCED PROVIDER	TRUE CONTRAINDICATION
• Thyroid conditions (Hashimoto's disease, hypothyroidism, thyroid nodules) and the use of thyroid hormone replacement* • Hormone replacement therapy • Polycystic ovarian syndrome (PCOS) • Most thyroid cancers* (papillary, follicular, Hürthle cell) • Gallbladder removal • Elevated pancreatic enzymes (not due to pancreatitis) • Irritable bowel syndrome (IBS) and related conditions* • History of pancreatitis*	• Type 1 diabetes* • Children and adolescents	• Medullary thyroid carcinoma (MTC) • Multiple endocrine neoplasia type 2 (MEN2)

Thyroid Conditions, MTC, and MEN2

The only absolute contraindication of taking a GLP-1 medication is a personal or first-degree family history of medullary thyroid carcinoma (MTC), which is a rare type of thyroid cancer that accounts for less than 2 percent of all thyroid cancers. MTC is associated with a genetic condition called multiple endocrine neoplasia type 2 (MEN2). Early mice studies showed an increase of medullary thyroid carcinoma in those on GLP-1 medications compared with those who were taking a placebo. It's important to note that this result has not been reproduced in humans. Still, it needs to be mentioned as a contraindication because of the results from the animal studies. That said, having a history of any other type of thyroid cancer (papillary, follicular, Hürthle cell carcinoma, etc.) is *not* a contraindication to taking a GLP-1. The same goes if you have thyroid nodules, hypothyroidism, or Hashimoto's, or take thyroid hormone replacement.

Pancreatitis

Pancreatitis is a serious condition that involves inflammation of the pancreas, and because GLP-1s act on the pancreas, it's understandable that patients with a history of pancreatitis have concerns that the medication may cause a relapse. The connection between GLP-1s and pancreatitis is drawn mostly from early research involving the Gila monster's venom (which caused pancreatitis in its prey and inspired early drug development). However, GLP-1 medications stimulate insulin release—but only when blood sugar levels are elevated. This targeted action makes it unlikely for the medication to lead to pancreatitis.

In real-world use, pancreatitis as a side effect of GLP-1s is very rare. It tends to occur in patients who have other risk factors for pancreatitis. Here's how many providers consider the risks of pancreatitis with the benefits of GLP-1 medications.

- If you've previously had documented pancreatitis caused by a GLP-1, the general recommendation is to avoid these medications.
- If your pancreatitis was unrelated to GLP-1 use, the situation is more nuanced. You may still be a candidate but only after careful discussion with an experienced and knowledgeable provider.

It's worth noting that pancreatitis is not subtle. It typically presents with severe and acute abdominal pain, nausea, and vomiting that require hospitalization, frequently in the intensive care unit. That is, if the above didn't happen, you didn't have pancreatitis.

IBS and Related Conditions

Many patients with IBS worry that GLP-1s will make their symptoms worse. But in practice, what we often see is the opposite. That's because GLP-1s tend to reduce your intake of highly processed, inflammatory foods, which are common triggers for IBS symptoms.

Within the first week or two of treatment, patients often notice improvements in their digestion, skin clarity, and even blood pressure. These changes occur too fast to be attributed to weight loss alone; they're more likely the result of reduced exposure to the high-sugar, high-fat, highly rewarding foods that trigger inflammation and gut issues. It's a chain reaction.

That said, if you have IBS or another gastrointestinal condition, it's important to go slow with increasing your dose of a GLP-1 and work closely with your provider. But these medications aren't off the table; for many patients, they're part of the solution.

Type 1 Diabetes

GLP-1 medications were designed for people with type 2 diabetes—but what about those with type 1 diabetes? Type 1 diabetes is caused by the body's inability to produce insulin, which means that GLP-1s, which stimulate the body to secrete insulin that it has already made, aren't useful for increasing insulin levels. That doesn't mean they're off the table.

In fact, I've had many patients with type 1 diabetes who struggle with appetite regulation, weight gain from insulin use, and uncontrolled glucose levels. For them, GLP-1s can provide life-changing benefits: reduced cravings, greater satiety, and lower insulin requirements. Their blood sugar level often becomes more stable, and they lose weight in a way they've never been able to before.

But this approach requires extremely careful management. If insulin doses aren't adjusted to account for decreased food intake and improved insulin sensitivity, the patient is at risk of developing severe hypoglycemia (low blood sugar). Anyone with type 1 diabetes using a GLP-1 should be closely followed by an experienced endocrinologist who can help adjust the dosage of insulin appropriately.

Polycystic Ovarian Syndrome (PCOS)

GLP-1s can be a powerful tool for patients with polycystic ovarian syndrome (PCOS). Despite what the name suggests, PCOS isn't really about having ovarian cysts. In fact, many people with PCOS don't have any at all; what are often labeled as cysts on a pelvic ultrasound are actually immature ovarian follicles, undeveloped eggs that haven't matured. Surprising, right? The real underlying issue in PCOS is hormonal, specifically, elevated levels of androgens such as testosterone, a condition called hyperandrogenemia.

This hormonal imbalance often results in symptoms such as hirsutism (thick, dark, coarse hair on the chin, chest, or other areas), acne, and scalp hair thinning or loss. But there's also a deeper metabolic connection. Elevated testosterone contributes to the buildup of visceral fat—the fat that surrounds your internal organs. And visceral fat is closely linked with insulin resistance, which in turn can worsen hormone levels. It's a cycle: More insulin resistance leads to more androgens, which leads to more insulin resistance.

This is where GLP-1s can help. They reduce insulin resistance, lower visceral fat, and help break the vicious metabolic-hormonal cycle at the heart of PCOS. In this context, GLP-1s don't just support weight loss; they target some of the root causes of PCOS itself.

CAMELIA'S STORY

I have a family history of PCOS and have struggled with the condition for as long as I can remember. I rarely got my period, was diagnosed as prediabetic, and dealt with constant weight fluctuations, water retention, acne, excess body hair, hair thinning, brain fog, fatigue, and anxiety. As a young girl, these symptoms were overwhelming. I saw countless doctors, and every single one told me that my levels were "normal" and I should just go on birth control to regulate my cycle.

I eventually did go on the Pill. My body changed, and it felt foreign to me. I decided to try the holistic route: I saw a nutritionist, cut out dairy products and gluten, took every single supplement under the sun, and did weekly acupuncture. I was lifting weights, eating healthy, and doing everything I could to find balance while navigating college and my early twenties. Some symptoms slightly improved, but I still didn't have periods—and I could not keep up with all of it. I was ready to give up. Maybe that was just how I was supposed to feel.

I still remember the day I found Dr. Salas and felt a glimpse of hope. I told my mom, "Please, just one more doctor—then I will surrender." I had a really good gut feeling about her.

She recommended starting tirzepatide, and a little bit over a year later, I am down thirty pounds, my symptoms are under control, and most important, I now have a regular period every month. I'm currently on the lowest dose for maintenance.

To say this medication changed my life is an understatement. At twenty-six, I finally feel like I have my confidence and spark back. I just wish I'd had access to it sooner—it would have saved me years of struggle.

Other Considerations: Life Stage, Hormones, and Age

When it comes to GLP-1 therapy, context matters. Your stage of life, hormonal landscape, age, and daily routines can all influence how your body responds to treatment—and what kind of support you might need along the way. In the following sections, we'll explore how factors such as adolescence, pregnancy, perimenopause, and lifestyle choices can shape your GLP-1 experience and what adjustments might help you stay on track.

Are You Trying to Conceive, Pregnant, or Breastfeeding?

There is one conversation I have all the time: Patients come to me excited—eager to finally lose the weight that's been holding them back but also just as eager to start or grow their family. And I understand both of those desires deeply. Those two goals don't have to compete—but using GLP-1s to get your body to a healthier place *before* conception is ideal. In chapter 1, I touched on how certain epigenetic changes can be passed down to future generations. Simply put, your prepregnancy weight matters—both for you and for your baby. Achieving a healthier weight and improved metabolic markers makes pregnancy safer for you, and it gives your future child a better chance at lifelong good health.

Fertility also tends to improve, as GLP-1s help reduce inflammation and insulin resistance, especially in patients with conditions such as PCOS. Male obesity has an equally negative impact on fertility. In many cases, GLP-1 treatment helps patients, both male and female, conceive naturally after months or even years of fertility challenges.

What does the timeline for taking GLP-1s look like if you are trying to conceive? It's generally recommended to postpone pregnancy until after you've reached your fat loss goal and then, ideally, take two to three months to gradually taper off the medication before trying to conceive. This gives you time to get more comfortable with the new eating habits that you've developed while on the medication. It also gives your body time to recalibrate before it is flooded with hormones again, ensuring a smooth transition to pregnancy for both you and your baby.

If pregnancy happens unexpectedly while on treatment, we typically stop the medication out of precaution. We want to be sure that the baby is getting enough nutrients. But every situation is different, and we always weigh the benefits and risks based on your medical history.

When it comes to breastfeeding and GLP-1 medications, the available data is extremely limited. In one small study involving semaglutide, the medication was not detected in human breast milk. Another study found that GLP-1 does not appear to transfer into breast milk in humans, although it did in animal models, specifically mice.

One proposed reason for this apparent safety is its molecular size: GLP-1 receptor agonists are large peptide molecules, likely too large to pass into breast milk in clinically meaningful amounts. Even if trace amounts did transfer, they would likely be degraded by the infant's digestive enzymes before absorption. That said, because pregnant and lactating individuals are routinely excluded from clinical trials, I approach this situation with caution and careful individual assessment. In my practice, decisions are made case by case, balancing maternal benefits with the lack of definitive safety data.

Perimenopause and Menopause

Perimenopause and menopause cause hormonal shifts that can translate to increased central adiposity and a loss of lean muscle mass. Many patients in midlife come to me and tell me, "Nothing I used to do works anymore." They're exercising more, eating better than ever, and still watching the scale climb. Sound familiar?

It's not just in your head; hormonal changes during perimenopause and menopause can drastically alter your body composition, metabolism, and fat distribution, especially around the abdomen. Women between the ages of forty and sixty-five accumulate, on average, 1.5 pounds per year, due largely to these hormonal changes. As their estrogen level declines, women often notice more weight accumulating around the midsection and a gradual loss of muscle, which can slow their metabolism and make it harder to maintain their weight, even with healthy habits. You may also experience symptoms such as mood shifts, low libido, poor sleep, and low energy—and while these are often chalked up to menopause alone, they're deeply connected to the metabolic and hormonal shifts that are happening under the surface.

GLP-1s can be a powerful tool during this time of life—not just for weight loss but for improving many overlapping symptoms. I've had patients in their late forties who came to my office for weight concerns and then experienced unexpected improvements in their energy, mood, and even sexual wellness after treatment began. In those cases, the medication helped resolve physical and emotional symptoms that had been dismissed for years.

GLP-1s can also be used safely alongside hormone replacement therapy (HRT). The two don't interact negatively; the decision to start one before the other or to begin both at the same time will depend on a patient's preference or acuity of symptoms. If it's unclear whether your symptoms stem more from weight gain or hormonal shifts, we often begin with a GLP-1 to address insulin resistance and inflammation and then see how your symptoms change.

A COOL PERK OF FAT LOSS

Excess fat acts like insulation, trapping heat and making it harder for your body to regulate its temperature. For many women in perimenopause or menopause, this can worsen their hot flashes, night sweats, and overall discomfort. One benefit of fat loss that you might not have considered is improved temperature regulation. As their fat mass decreases, many patients using GLP-1s report fewer hot flashes and less overheating at night. Definitely a welcome bonus!

Age Considerations: Children, Teens, Young Adults, and Older Adults

While this book speaks primarily to adults navigating their own care, many readers are also parents—and obesity is often a family issue genetically, behaviorally, and environmentally. It's not unusual for patients to ask, "Is this something that could help my child, too?" The answer is often "yes"—so let's take a closer look at how GLP-1s can be used across different life stages.

Children

GLP-1 medications are currently FDA approved for treating type 2 diabetes in children ten years and older and for weight loss in children twelve and up. That said, it may be appropriate to use GLP-1s off-label in younger children under the care of an experienced provider—particularly in cases of severe obesity or where there are obesity-related health concerns.

In my clinical practice, I've worked with several prepubescent children. The most important consideration for children who haven't reached puberty is maintaining their growth. We keep a close eye on the child's height, measuring it at every visit, and always use the lowest effective dose. If the child shows any signs of stalled growth, we stop the medication immediately to enable a catch-up growth spurt. Once they've reached their final height, we can revisit the idea of treatment again if it's still appropriate. Success with GLP-1 therapy for these patients is all about finding the right balance between supporting a healthy weight and preserving a healthy growth pattern.

With younger patients, the conversation is more nuanced. GLP-1s work best when paired with healthy eating and physical activity, because it can be tempting for the patients—or their parents—to view the medication as a quick fix. That's why I always stress that GLP-1 therapy is a clinical intervention to support long-term health.

In these cases, partnership with parents is key. Everyone involved needs to understand that this is not cosmetic weight loss; the goal is not simply to "get thin," but to reduce long-term health risks and improve quality of life. When used thoughtfully and responsibly, GLP-1s can be life-changing for young people—but they work best when framed as just one part of a broader strategy that includes nutrition, movement, emotional support, and education.

Young Adults

What about college students and young adults? For many people in this age group, weight gain can come on gradually (as in the form of the dreaded "Freshman 15"). This is often triggered by lifestyle changes, stress, less structured routines, or a shift away from their past activity level or sports. For a patient in this age group who has been persistently struggling with weight, GLP-1s can be an option; however, there are some lifestyle factors to take into consideration (more on that in a moment).

Many young adults respond well to treatment; they often see noticeable results at lower doses and with fewer side effects compared with older adults. Their bodies may be more responsive to changes in insulin and appetite signaling, which can lead to quicker improvements in weight and metabolic health, especially if they're motivated and ready to make lifestyle changes. But adherence can be more challenging in this age group, particularly if priorities such as school and social life are competing for their attention.

College and Social Drinking

For many college students and young adults, social drinking is a large part of their social landscape, and that's where things can get tricky. GLP-1s slow down digestion and reduce appetite, which can make it harder to stay hydrated and tolerate alcohol. Add binge drinking into the mix (and the late-night snacks that usually come with it), and you've got a perfect storm: nausea, vomiting, digestive issues, dehydration, and sometimes even hospital visits.

I like to have an extremely honest conversation with my patients who partake in frequent social drinking. If they know that that's a part of their life that they're realistically not going to give up, we can try a GLP-1 on a low dose and see how they tolerate it. But if a patient wants to escalate to a higher dose to see fat loss results more quickly, alcohol often has to come off the table—at least for a while. It becomes a matter of evaluating priorities: Are they in a season of life where they're ready and willing to focus on their health? Or is this just not the right time to introduce a major lifestyle change?

This is an example of why a personalized approach is so important; it's not always an easy "yes" or "no" for each patient. It is crucial that providers help their patients make an informed choice that reflects their goals and reality.

Older Adults

If you're wondering whether there's an upper age limit for starting a GLP-1 medication, there's good news: There really isn't. I've had patients start treatment well into their seventies and eighties. It's never too late to take meaningful steps toward better health, improved mobility, and greater quality of life.

That said, certain precautions are important when prescribing GLP-1s in older adults. Sarcopenia, the age-related loss of muscle mass and strength, is already a concern in this population. GLP-1 therapies, while effective for weight loss and metabolic improvement, can potentially worsen muscle loss if not managed carefully. That's why ensuring adequate protein intake, encouraging resistance training, and monitoring body composition are essential in this age group.

Additionally, it's important to assess kidney function before initiating therapy. Some degree of chronic kidney disease is common in older adults, and impaired renal function may affect both the safety and tolerability of certain GLP-1 medications.

Always speak with your doctor about your individual health status and potential risks. But if you are medically eligible, age alone should never be a barrier to treatment.

Committing to a Long-Term Treatment

How long a patient will need to take a GLP-1 medication varies from person to person. The length of your treatment will depend on why you're taking the medication, what your goals are, and how your body responds to the medication.

Understanding this from the start can make a big difference. Knowing that GLP-1s are often a long-term therapy helps you approach your treatment from the right perspective. When you realize that you're managing a chronic condition—not trying to "fix" yourself overnight—it becomes easier to stick with the process and stay grounded through ups and downs.

For patients with chronic obesity or overweight, yes, GLP-1 medications are generally a long-term or even lifelong tool. That said, the goal is always to use the *lowest effective dose* to maintain results and minimize side effects. (I'll go into more detail about dosage and maintenance in chapter 8.) With the right lifestyle adjustments, especially of nutrition and exercise, the majority of patients can taper down to a much lower dose over time, use the medication intermittently, or even, for a few, stop taking it altogether, especially if they haven't struggled with weight for most of their life (in other words, someone with a "Sudden Shift" or "Life Event That Changes Everything" weight story). The dose and duration of your GLP-1 therapy are dynamic, not fixed. The more you do to support your body when you take these medications, the more options you'll have for adjusting how much you need to take and how long your treatment will last.

If the possibility of using a GLP-1 medication long term gives you pause, you are not alone. Many of my patients have the same reaction when they learn that GLP-1 therapy may not be a one-and-done solution. If this is you, I encourage you to remember that excess weight is not a cosmetic issue or a problem to be solved. If you keep thinking of GLP-1 treatment only through the lens of "fixing" how you look, it makes sense that you'd wonder how long you must take it before you're "done."

I want to lead you away from this perspective. Obesity is a chronic, multifactorial medical condition. A chronic disease is not curable and can only be controlled. Think of obesity as being like hypertension or high cholesterol, and GLP-1s as being like a diuretic or a statin. If your body naturally struggles with regulating weight due to hormonal, genetic, or metabolic factors, stopping GLP-1 medication might bring back the same challenges, just as someone with hypertension who stops their medication might see their blood pressure rise again.

Don't frame GLP-1 therapy as being dependent on a medication forever; think of it as a way to give your body the support it needs for as long as it needs it—without shame or stigma. We don't ask people with asthma how long they plan to use an inhaler or expect people with high cholesterol to "will" their levels to drop after a few months. This is no different.

MY STORY

For a real-life example of how some people can use GLP-1 therapy temporarily, I want to share my own experience on a GLP-1 medication. My weight story falls under "The Sudden Shift." I had never struggled with weight, nor did I have a strong family history of obesity on either side of my family. I had an active lifestyle and had enjoyed weightlifting since my early twenties.

My life journey (and years of medical training) led me to have my daughters at ages thirty-eight and thirty-nine years. During my first pregnancy, I gained a whopping seventy pounds. I remember my OB pleading with me to watch my weight during every prenatal visit. Just five months after giving birth, I was pregnant again. That time, I was more mindful and gained only thirty pounds. But by the time I delivered my second daughter, I was in my early forties—carrying thirty extra pounds, raising two kids under two years of age, and beginning to experience the hormonal shifts of perimenopause.

To be honest, in those early years I didn't prioritize weight loss. I gave myself grace. I was exhausted and focused mainly on getting through that chapter of motherhood. Losing weight was not a top priority for me, and I didn't beat myself up about it.

Eventually, I started semaglutide. I didn't feel ashamed about needing support and didn't feel that I needed to "earn" the medication route by exhausting every other option first. I trusted the science, and I gave myself permission to use a tool that made sense for me and my situation.

Truthfully, my experience with my patients was why I was able to make that decision without shame or hesitation. Over the years, they've shown me what most of us were never taught: that weight isn't about willpower and needing help isn't a personal failure.

That knowledge protected me from the guilt and self-blame so many people experience, and I hope the knowledge I'm sharing in this book will do the same for you. After about twenty-four weeks of treatment, I was back to a healthy weight. I gradually stopped the medication and haven't needed it since—but if that ever changes, I wouldn't hesitate to start again.

Your Story, Your Solution

By now you've probably gathered that the answer to the question of whether you are a candidate for GLP-1s is more often than not "yes." These medications were once thought to be helpful for only the most extreme or clear-cut cases—but our understanding of them has evolved. We now know that GLP-1s can benefit a wide range of patients with different body types, histories, and needs.

But that doesn't mean this is a one-size-fits-all solution. Every patient's story is different, and there are many important variables to consider: your medical history, your goals, your timeline, your stage of life, and your overall health picture.

Whether you've struggled with weight since childhood, gained it unexpectedly in midlife, or simply feel that your body no longer responds to the things that used to work—this next chapter could be the start of something different. It will help you find the foundation for creating the right support and strategy. You'll be equipped not just to start this therapy but to make it work for *you*.

CHAPTER 4

The Road Starts Here: Finding the Right Provider and Getting Your Prescription

I hope chapter 3 left you feeling not only informed but genuinely excited about the life-changing potential of GLP-1 medications. Now you're standing at the beginning of the path ahead—but what's the first step? Where do you even start?

The current landscape of GLP-1s can feel like a maze—or sometimes a minefield. The demand for them is sky-high, and as a result, the business of providing them has exploded. There's a lot of noise to sort through, and not all of it is coming from trustworthy sources.

This landscape is why this chapter is one of the most important in the book. It includes everything you should know after deciding to pursue treatment with a GLP-1. It's the tool kit that will help you build a solid foundation for your GLP-1 journey even before you take your first dose. Whether you're working with a top-tier obesity specialist or navigating a telehealth platform, by the end of this chapter you'll know exactly how to choose the right provider, what questions to ask, and red flags to watch out for. Feeling confident that you have the right guidance and care is the first step to success—let's make sure you start off strong.

Choosing the Right Provider

After deciding to start GLP-1 therapy, the next step is choosing the right provider. Starting GLP-1 therapy isn't just about getting the medication; it's about getting the right care. The quality of your experience will depend heavily on the knowledge and experience of your provider. You deserve more than a rushed prescription and a wave out the door; you deserve a reliable expert—someone who understands the nuances of these medications, takes time to understand your history, and helps guide your success.

Ideally, that partner is a provider who has real, extensive experience treating patients with GLP-1s. The safety and efficacy of these medications are directly tied to the expertise of the provider prescribing them. In simple terms, if you want the best results with the fewest side effects, you need someone who knows what they're doing, someone with a track record of success.

Traditionally, endocrinologists were considered the go-to specialists for weight and metabolism concerns. As part of our training, we study how weight gain affects the body, how hormones interact, and how conditions such as diabetes develop. But endocrinology alone doesn't fully encompass the complexity of obesity. That's why in 2011, the specialty of obesity medicine was formally established.

Physicians who are board certified in obesity medicine have advanced, targeted training in treating obesity as a chronic, multifactorial disease. Unlike general endocrinology, which covers a wide range of hormone-related conditions, obesity medicine focuses on the science of body weight regulation and the dozens of interrelated factors that influence it, including genetics, neurohormonal signaling, food addiction, gut microbiota, medications, mental health, sleep, and lifestyle behaviors.

To earn this certification, providers must complete extensive continuing education and demonstrate competency in four core pillars of treatment—nutrition, physical activity, behavioral support, and pharmacotherapy—on top of passing a rigorous board exam. They're also trained to recognize how root causes such as chronic stress, insulin resistance, and disrupted sleep contribute to weight gain and to craft personalized treatment plans.

This makes a certified obesity medicine specialist uniquely qualified to guide you through GLP-1 therapy. These providers understand the truth about obesity and will look at every aspect of your life and lifestyle. They can individualize dosing strategies, prevent unnecessary side effects, monitor lean muscle mass, and integrate life changes to maximize long-term results.

As of 2025, there are just under 10,000 certified obesity medicine specialists in the United States. With applications for the obesity board exam more than tripling in the past five years, obesity medicine has become the fastest-growing medical specialty.

It's good news that more and more doctors want to join this field, but right now, you'll still need to do a bit of detective work to find someone you can really trust to lead you on your journey safely and successfully. Don't worry; we're going to go over how to do just that.

What I Learned Once I Had Time to Listen

Not every provider has the time or freedom to deliver the care they want to. I know this because, for years, I was one of them. I didn't learn most of what I know about treating obesity during the fourteen years of training I went through to become an endocrinologist; I learned it after I opened my clinic in 2019.

As young doctors, we're trained to follow strict protocols, and our time is scheduled down to the minute. During my outpatient rotations, I was given fifteen minutes for each appointment regardless of whether the patient was new or returning. I would try to take notes between patients, but there was no time and I'd quickly get behind. When I asked my attending physician for advice, she suggested that I type up notes as the patient was speaking. But I couldn't—and I didn't. How could I expect a patient to open up and trust me if my mind was on my notes instead of their story and my eyes were fixed on a screen? How could I possibly understand what they needed if I didn't give them the space to tell me?

That experience taught me one of the most important lessons in medicine: If you give people the space to speak, open up, and be vulnerable, they'll tell you exactly what they need.

We are set up to fail as physicians when we are not given the freedom to practice medicine as we see fit. It wasn't until I started my own practice and had the agency to spend an hour or more with my patients that I truly began to understand obesity. I will be forever grateful to my greatest teachers: my patients.

In chapter 1, we explored how obesity is a far more complex condition than most of us were led to believe. But weight loss? It's even more complicated. For decades, we equated success with a number on the scale, using BMI as our guide. We praised weight loss without asking what exactly had been lost—or why the weight had been there in the first place. GLP-1 medications have changed the way I see all of this. They've

> helped us understand how appetite is regulated, how the brain processes reward, and how fat, not just weight, is lost.
>
> I share these experiences because I want you to know that if you've ever felt dismissed or rushed through an appointment, it's not your fault—and it may not even be your doctor's. It's the system's. But you deserve a provider who listens, and you'll benefit the most from one, too.
>
> I hope that the advice in this chapter will help you find such a provider.

What to Look for When Choosing Your Provider

Finding the right provider starts with asking the right questions. These questions will give you a strong sense of how knowledgeable and experienced the provider is and whether they're the right fit for you.

Is the Doctor Board Certified? In What Specialty or Specialties?

For the reasons just discussed, it is ideal for your provider to be board certified in obesity medicine. They'll have the most experience working with patients who have obesity or overweight. The easiest way to find a board-certified obesity medicine physician is through the American Board of Obesity Medicine's website (abom.org). Enter your zip code, and it will generate a list of certified providers in your area.

Your second-best bet will be an endocrinologist. Many newer endocrinologists are increasingly well versed in obesity treatment, though not all of them have hands-on experience with GLP-1s. Be sure to ask about their experience.

Your third option is a board-certified primary care or family medicine physician.

The Road Starts Here

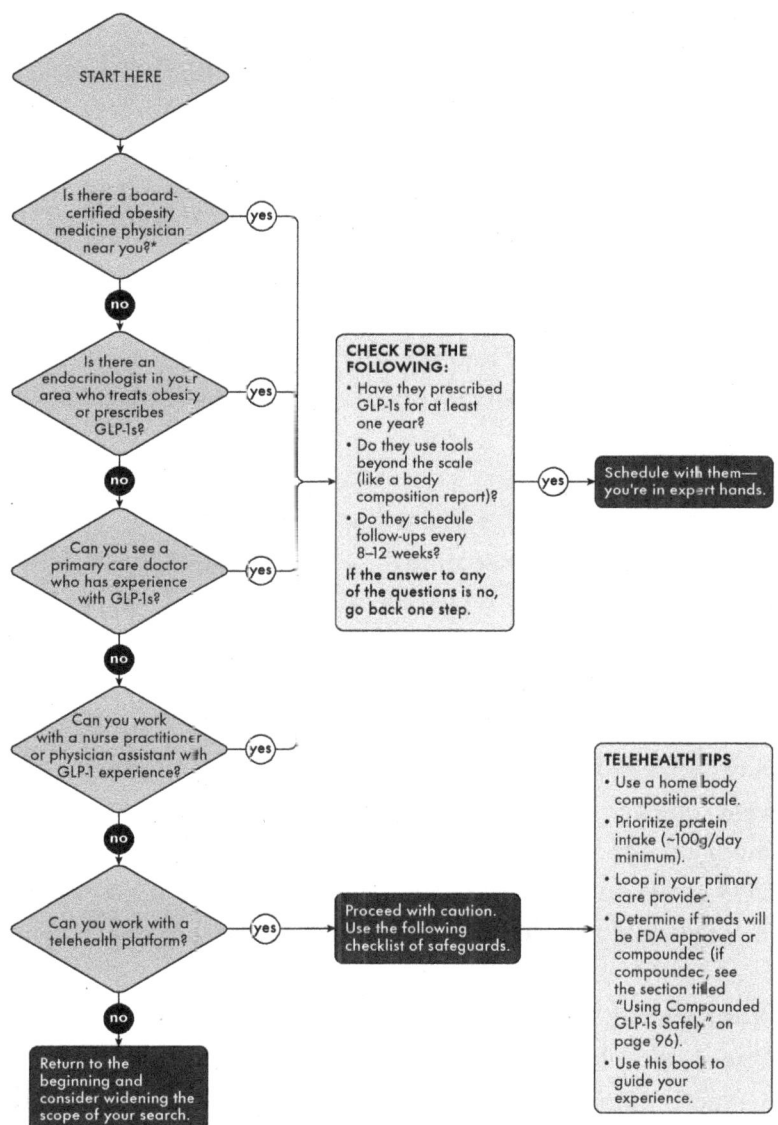

*Check abom.org for certified providers.

Since there are not enough physicians and specialists certified in obesity medicine, you can also benefit from ancillary providers such as nurse practitioners and physician's assistants. Many of them may have more experience with prescribing GLP-1 medications than a more generalized primary care provider, and their expertise will be valuable.

Remember, many providers are still learning about GLP-1 therapy. Obesity medicine and GLP-1 medications are new territory for most doctors, and they're figuring things out as they go along. Depending on where you live and what kind of access you have, the ideal provider may not be available to you. (If that's the case, the next best thing is already in your hands—and you're reading it right now.)

Does the Provider Have Experience Prescribing GLP-1 Medications?

The easiest way to know if your provider is an experienced prescriber is to call the provider's office and ask. Never assume that a doctor prescribes GLP-1 medications, even if their specialty could indicate that.

I also recommend asking how long they have prescribed it. You want someone who has prescribed a GLP-1 medication for a minimum of one year. To really gain experience in prescribing a GLP-1, a provider needs to see a patient a couple of times before they can truly understand how the medications work.

What Metrics Do They Use to Diagnose Obesity and Track Progress?

A simple litmus test to determine whether a provider has experience with GLP-1s is to ask if they use any measurement beyond the scale—such as body composition analysis—to diagnose obesity and track progress. If they don't, that's a red flag. Usually, this information will be advertised on their business website. If not, ask when calling to make an appointment.

How Often Do They Schedule Follow-up Visits for Patients on GLP-1s?

Follow-ups are a *must*. If a provider gives you a prescription and doesn't plan to see you again, it's a red flag. It indicates that they have no idea how these drugs work and that they may be more interested in increasing the number of patients that GLP-1 prescriptions can bring in than providing quality care to each one. Ideally you want to be seen every eight to twelve weeks to monitor your progress and adjust your dosage as needed. In some cases, more frequent visits may be appropriate. On the other hand, weekly visits, especially those focused solely on weighing in, are typically a feature of med spas, not medical practices. It generally takes four to six weeks to begin seeing meaningful changes in body composition.

Many of the answers to these questions can be found on the provider's website or by making a call to the office. If the provider is experienced with treating obesity by using GLP-1 therapy, the front desk should have these answers quickly—a green flag.

NANCY'S STORY

I've always been a very active person. I played soccer in middle school and in college. I wouldn't say I was superfit, but I was active and healthy enough. When I got pregnant in my early twenties, I was around 125 pounds. The last time I saw the scale before my son was born, I was just two pounds shy of 200. That was when my problem with weight began.

From that point forward, the scale kept creeping up year after year. I could see it and feel it. I returned to the gym, worked with a personal trainer, and even went back to playing soccer. My activity level was there, but I just wasn't seeing the numbers on the scale go down. I struggled with weight from my early twenties until my late thirties, when I started my GLP-1 journey.

I felt excited and well prepared because of the consultation I had with my doctor. My doctor explained what to expect, what might go wrong, and how to fix it if it did. In my nearly four years of treatment, I experienced a few side effects here and there, including brief hair loss, occasional lightheadedness, and feeling sick to my stomach. That might sound bad, but I don't believe I had a negative experience overall because I understood the "why" behind each symptom, and, more important, I knew how to manage them.

My biggest advice? Do your research on the medicine and your doctor.

What About Telehealth Platforms?

In today's world, you can't scroll on social media or walk through a city without seeing ads for telemedicine platforms offering GLP-1s. These services are springing up all over the place, and they make getting started with GLP-1 therapy feel incredibly easy. With just a short questionnaire, many will ship the medication straight to your door. Given the shortage of experienced providers and the lack of access in rural areas, telemedicine has a place. But while access to them is easy, support for them is often minimal. Most of these companies don't assess body composition, review your full medical history, or provide personalized guidance. Many offer only compounded medications, which may be cheaper than brand-name meds, but remember, they aren't permitted under current FDA guidelines and could signal a red flag when offered routinely.

If you're using one of these platforms, you may feel as though you're navigating this journey alone. And in many ways, you are. But once you're armed with all the knowledge and tools you need for success, you can take ownership of your experience and achieve a great outcome.

Tips for Better Outcomes with Telehealth
- **Get a home body composition scale.** It doesn't need to be top of the line, just consistent. Tracking changes in your muscle mass and fat is crucial. (See chapter 5 to learn how.)
- **Pay special attention to your protein intake.** If you can't measure your body composition, hitting your daily protein goal can help ensure that you're losing fat, not muscle. (In my clinical experience, about 100 grams per day is the minimum; I'll go deeper into this in chapter 6.)
- **Loop in your primary care provider.** Let them know that you're accessing GLP-1 therapy through a telehealth platform. Having another set of eyes on your journey will make it safer.

What to Expect at Your First Appointment

At last—the appointment you've been waiting for is here. Your first visit with your provider marks the beginning of a new chapter in your health journey. Are you excited? You should be! I certainly am.

This first appointment is an important opportunity for your provider to learn about you and your history, and for you as the patient to learn what the path ahead may look like. Here are some things to expect during your first appointment so you can go in prepared. (You can also find a quick-reference appointment checklist on page 230.)

1. **A vulnerable conversation with your provider:** Your provider will want to dig into your personal history with weight and

health history, so it's best to come prepared with answers that are as detailed as possible. If you're going the telehealth route or you think your provider won't prioritize this kind of conversation, it's even more important to take some time beforehand to think about your responses. Going through your history is important for helping you understand the patterns that may be contributing to your weight history and the factors that have been beyond your control. Here's what to think about in advance.

- **Your weight story:** When did your weight story begin? What diets, programs, or routines have you tried? What worked, and what didn't? What's the heaviest you've been (outside of pregnancy), and what weight felt most sustainable for you?
- **Your family history:** Consider your family's relationship with weight. Has anyone else struggled with their weight? Think critically about your answer; perhaps your family members are not overweight, but they maintain restrictive behaviors or require conscious effort to remain at their goal weight.
- **Your medications:** Bring a list of all medications you are currently taking, including names, dosages, and any past weight-related treatments you've tried.
- **Your lifestyle:** Be honest and specific about your eating and exercise habits. What do you typically eat in a day? Do you skip breakfast? What does a week of movement look like for you?
- **Your relationship with food:** Do you eat for stress relief, boredom, anxiety, or celebration? Do you feel in control or out of control around food? Have you ever struggled with disordered eating? Knowing some of the subconscious motivations behind your eating habits will help you on your GLP-1 journey.
- **Your alcohol use:** How often do you drink alcohol? Is it social, habitual, or a form of stress relief? Do

you subconsciously anticipate a reward or an effect when you have a drink, even if it's just to "loosen up" or "relax"? (If so, your relationship to alcohol will change as GLP-1s affect your reward systems; I'll discuss this more in the next chapter.)

- **Your hormone history:** If you are a woman, when was your first period? Have you had irregular cycles, tried to conceive, experienced pregnancy or postpartum changes? Have you been diagnosed with PCOS or any other hormonal issue?
- **Your family dynamics:** Do your children struggle with their weight? What's the weight story of their other parent? These factors provide insights into potential genetic and environmental contributors.

2. **Bloodwork and metabolic panels:** Your provider may order labs to assess your baseline metabolic health and rule out any potential contributing factors or underlying conditions.

3. **Body composition assessment:** Ideally, your provider will measure more than your weight and BMI. A DEXA scan or professional, in-office BIA scale assessment can provide critical insight into your body composition and can be more accurate and thorough than the consumer versions designed for home use.

4. **Custom treatment plan:** Based on the information you shared and after a thorough physical exam that hopefully included a body composition assessment, your provider will discuss if a GLP-1 is an option for you. If they decide that it is, you and your provider will determine which one would be a good place for you to start. In the vast majority of cases, unless there's a specific reason to wait for lab results, you should expect to walk out with a prescription. In my office, you may even be able to get your first dose at your first appointment.

You've waited long enough! Ideally, your doctor will plan to see you every eight to twelve weeks or so for follow-up appointments.

The above should give you a clear picture of what to expect at your first appointment. Hopefully, you'll walk away feeling confident in the provider you've chosen and supported in taking the next step.

> ### When Your Provider Isn't a Good Fit
>
> What if you did your research to pick the right doctor or provider, but realized after your first visit that they might not be the right one *for you*?
>
> Kudos to you for following your gut. You want a provider you see eye to eye with, who you feel connected to, and who makes you feel comfortable. Granted, you might need a few office visits to feel this way. But if from day one, you don't feel heard, seen, or comfortable, it's better to change providers now rather than later—although you can explore other options at any point in your GLP-1 journey.

Which GLP-1 Is Right for You?

We touched on the science behind GLP-1 medications in chapter 2. Now let's explore how your doctor decides which of the GLP-1 agonists on the market is best for you. While all GLP-1 receptor agonists work similarly in the body, they differ in a few important ways:

- Their FDA-approved uses (some are approved for treating type 2 diabetes, chronic weight management, or both)
- Dosing schedules (daily versus weekly injections)

- Side effect profiles and how well your body tolerates them
- Insurance coverage and medication access
- The dosage range, which can affect both a medication's effectiveness and how well your body tolerates it
- The active ingredient

There are three primary active ingredients used in GLP-1 therapies: **semaglutide, tirzepatide,** and **liraglutide.** Though there are only three core ingredients, there are six medications on the market. Why? Drugs with each of these ingredients are sold under two brand names: one approved for treating type 2 diabetes and another approved for chronic weight management. The use, dosage, and branding of the medication approved for type 2 diabetes and the one approved for weight management may differ, even if the active ingredient is the same. The following diagram will help you visualize how each active ingredient corresponds to its two FDA-approved versions.

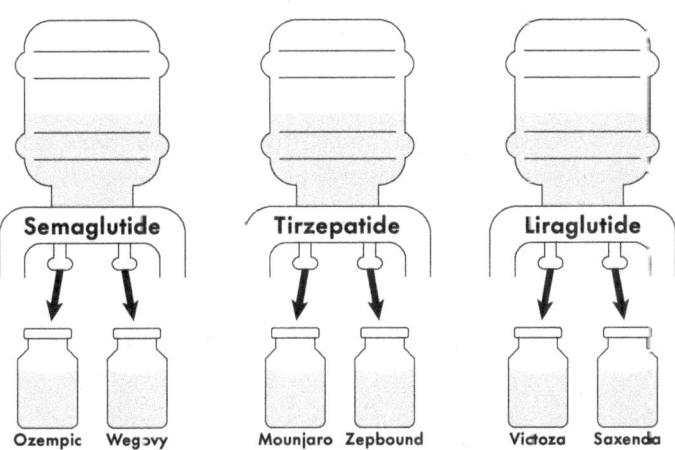

Now let's take a closer look at what you need to know about each active ingredient and what they might mean for you. As you review this information, please keep in mind that your doctor's choice of medication is not set in stone. Your doctor may adjust your prescription based on how you're responding or if access to a medication becomes an issue.

Semaglutide (Wegovy and Ozempic)

FDA Approvals
- Ozempic is FDA approved for type 2 diabetes.
- Wegovy is FDA approved for chronic weight management.

Why your doctor might choose it: At the time of writing, semaglutide remains the go-to GLP-1 for many providers, as it's the first drug that many feel comfortable prescribing. Ozempic may be preferred if you have diabetes. Wegovy is a strong choice for weight loss in nondiabetic patients because it can be taken at a higher dose, which is more effective for weight loss.

Dosing overview: Weekly injections of Ozempic start at a dose of 0.25 milligram and increase to 0.5 milligram, 1 milligram, and 2 milligrams (the maximum dose for the Ozempic pen). For Wegovy, doses are available at 0.25 milligram, 0.5 milligram, 1 milligram, 1.7 milligrams, and 2.4 milligrams (the maximum dose). At the time of writing this book, Wegovy is being studied at a 7.4-milligram dose.

Good to know: Semaglutide requires a slow, gradual increase in the dose, a process known as titration. Gradual titration reduces side effects but can delay noticeable weight loss. Some patients experience more nausea when taking semaglutides.

Tirzepatide (Zepbound and Mounjaro)

FDA Approvals
- Mounjaro is approved for type 2 diabetes.
- Zepbound is approved for chronic weight management.

Why your doctor might choose it: Tirzepatide can be more effective than semaglutide for weight loss and tends to be better tolerated.

Dosing overview: Weekly injections start at a dose of 2.5 milligrams and increase to 5 milligrams, 7.5 milligrams, 10 milligrams, 12.5 milligrams, and 15 milligrams (the maximum dose in both presentations of tirzepatide).

Good to know: Remember, tirzepatide is a dual agonist. It activates both GLP-1 and GIP receptors, which may be why you may see more weight loss than with semaglutide.

Liraglutide (Saxenda and Victoza)

FDA Approvals
- Victoza is approved for type 2 diabetes.
- Saxenda is approved for chronic weight management.

Why your doctor might choose it: Liraglutide is often used when access to newer GLP-1 medications is limited by cost or shortages. It also tends to be more widely covered by some insurance plans because it has spent more time on the market.

Dosing overview: Daily injections start at a dose of 0.6 milligram and increase to 1.2 milligrams, 1.8 milligrams, 2.4 milligrams, and 3 milligrams (the maximum dose).

Good to know: Weight loss results may be more modest than with semaglutide or tirzepatide. Because nausea can be more pronounced than with the GLP-1 medications that are taken weekly, titration to a higher dose happens more slowly. However, for the right patient and circumstances, liraglutide remains a valuable option.

THERAPEUTIC VERSUS SUBTHERAPEUTIC DOSES

If you're prescribed semaglutide or liraglutide, you will be asked to start with a subtherapeutic dose. A therapeutic dose of a medication means that you're taking an amount that will produce the desired effect (in this case, support significant weight loss and improve metabolic health), while a subtherapeutic dose is intended primarily to help your body adjust to a medication and may not spark big changes right away. But as with anything else in medicine, there are exceptions; some patients may lose weight even at smaller doses. You won't know how your body will respond until you start!

However, if you are taking tirzepatide, the starting 2.5 milligrams is a *therapeutic* dose. Some patients lose meaningful weight even at this first dose. Patients tend to tolerate tirzepatide better than semaglutide, which allowed Eli Lilly to design the starting dose (2.5 milligrams) to be therapeutic. Since side effects are milder at the therapeutic dose, there is no need to begin with a subtherapeutic dose.

What Happens at Home

Your success doesn't depend only on what happens in the provider's office; it also depends on what happens afterward, at home. There is a bit of "homework" involved, but I promise, it's the kind that will empower you to take ownership of your health. GLP-1 therapy is a team effort; your doctor helps guide the process, but your engagement and feedback are just as vital.

Here's a preview of a few things you can do between appointments to stay on track and support your progress from the very start. We'll cover many of these topics in more depth in part two of the book.

- **Tracking and accountability:** You'll be responsible for implementing new habits, tracking your symptoms and progress, and staying consistent with your follow-up appointments.
- **Body composition monitoring:** Invest in a home BIA scale to keep a closer eye on your body composition.
- **Lifestyle changes:** Get ready to focus significantly on your protein intake and weight training to help preserve your muscle mass—a crucial part of your success on GLP-1s. It's not just a "diet" or "exercise plan" for you to follow during treatment; it's a crucial way to support the medication, and it's part of your treatment plan. Period.
- **Ongoing communication:** Whether through follow-ups, check-ins, or questions that arise and need answers, staying in regular contact with your provider (or keeping personal records if using telehealth) will be important to staying on track.

Navigating the Cost and Why Your Health Is Worth It

Now let's talk about the uncomfortable truth: These medications are expensive, especially in the United States. And unfortunately, many insurance companies still make it extremely difficult to get them covered, even though so many people could benefit so greatly from them. If you're staring at the price tag and feeling discouraged, you're certainly not alone. But before you start talking yourself out of treatment, I want to gently encourage you to *reframe your thinking.*

So many of us have become accustomed to deprioritizing our health. We spend money on everything and everyone else before we consider spending on ourselves, especially when it comes to preventive, long-term health investments. But I want to emphasize that *you cannot put a price on what it feels like to be physically well.* To reduce your risk of disease. To move through the world feeling more confident and comfortable. To feel strong and healthy in your body.

You may have already spent years—and hundreds or thousands of dollars—chasing that fantasy. Think about all the diet books, cleanses, juice fasts, supplements, exercise programs, retreats, "boot camps," and cosmetic procedures intended to get your body to a point where you'd be happy with it. The saddest part is that for most people, none of those things actually works despite the cost.

GLP-1s are different. They are not a quick fix that may or may not stick; they are powerful medications backed by evidence. Many of my patients tell me that investing in this medication was the moment everything changed. For the first time, they stopped spending all their time, energy, and money trying to brute-force their way to "thin" and were able to begin healing their relationship with food and their bodies.

If you do this right, you'll never have to buy another diet book again; that is a promise I can make you. You'll also likely spend less on food, thanks to fewer cravings and smaller portion sizes. GLP-1 therapy is an investment in your future self. That said, I know that committing to GLP-1 therapy is not just about mindset; cost is a very real barrier for many. Here are a few ways to help make GLP-1 medications more financially accessible:

- **Manufacturer coupons:** Both pharmaceutical companies that produce GLP-1s (Novo Nordisk and Eli Lilly) offer significant savings through direct manufacturer coupons.

These can bring the cost down by hundreds of dollars per month, depending on your insurance status and income level.

- **Direct-to-patient pharmacy delivery programs:** Both Lilly and Novo Nordisk also offer pharmacy delivery programs that can sometimes reduce costs even more. For example, Lilly offers a lower-cost option for Zepbound that comes as a syringe kit and sells pen injectors at a reduced price.

Navigating Insurance Coverage

Navigating insurance coverage for GLP-1 medications can be one of the most frustrating parts of treatment. Here's what to expect and how to improve your chances of getting your prescription covered.

Start with a call to your insurance company to ask whether GLP-1 medications are covered and what documentation is required. In most cases, plans require prior authorization, which is a common but often challenging process. You'll likely need to submit documentation such as your BMI, qualifying diagnoses, and a history of previous treatment attempts. Be prepared for this to take anywhere from several days to weeks. Even then, initial requests are sometimes denied, so don't be discouraged. Many patients are approved on a second or even third try.

It's also worth noting that some providers opt out of this process entirely. Because it's so time and labor intensive and because demand is so high, some offices and clinics simply don't have the capacity to keep up. Ask in advance—if your provider doesn't handle it, you may be able to request a letter of medical necessity and submit the paperwork yourself or work with a pharmacy or third-party service that will handle the process on your behalf.

Using Compounded GLP-1s Safely

Let me be clear: As a board-certified physician, **I recommend using only FDA-approved GLP-1 medications.** These are the gold standard. Formulations such as Ozempic, Wegovy, and Zepbound undergo rigorous testing, consistent quality control, and ongoing FDA oversight. If they're accessible to you, they are unequivocally the safer and more reliable option.

That said, I also understand the financial reality: These medications are expensive, and not everyone will have insurance coverage or access. Hopefully, with time, prices will drop and access will improve, but until then, some patients may feel that they have no option but to use compounded GLP-1s. While I don't recommend it, if you're planning to use a compounded version anyway, it's critical that you do so as safely as possible.

Understand the Risks

As I covered in chapter 2, compounded GLP-1s are not FDA approved. They are made in pharmacies that blend or alter existing formulations and often use bulk-supplied pharmaceutical ingredients that may not have consistent potency, purity, or safety testing.

While they may seem like a bargain compared to the brand names, it's important to understand where that saving comes from: skipping the expensive steps of regulatory oversight, clinic trials, or quality standards that the FDA mandates for consistency, safety, and efficacy. As a result, compounded versions can carry real dangers, ranging from inaccurate dosing to unverified ingredients to long-term health risks. Still, if you're determined to move forward with compounded medication, here's how to do so safely.

Choose the Right Type of Pharmacy
There are two categories of compounding pharmacies:
- **503A pharmacies:** These are traditional compounding pharmacies that make a specific medication in response to a prescription for an individual patient. They are overseen by state pharmacy boards. While they are required to follow United States Pharmacopeia (USP) standards, they are not registered or regulated by the FDA.
- **503B outsourcing facilities:** These are more rigorously regulated and must be registered with the FDA. They are held to higher standards for sterility, quality control, and batch testing. They're allowed to produce larger batches of medication, often in anticipation of demand, and are required to undergo regular FDA inspections.

If you must use a compounded medication, choose one that comes from a 503B registered facility. You're far less likely to get something unsafe or inconsistently dosed.

Ask Questions About Your Compounded Medication
Before you decide on anything, ask your provider or pharmacy these questions.
- Is this medication from a 503B registered facility?
- Is there documentation of sterility and potency testing?
- Has the pharmacy been inspected by the FDA?
- What version of the active ingredient is being used, and how does it compare with the FDA-approved formulation?

Keep in mind that a legally compounded medication must differ from the commercial product in a clinically meaningful way to avoid infringing on the company's patent; make sure you know exactly how yours differs from the brand name.

If your provider can't or won't answer these questions or if you don't feel confident in their answers, it's best to look elsewhere. Some med spas, online clinics, and GLP-1 mills source their injections from unregulated pharmacies or even make them in-house, and patients don't have any idea where they're coming from. Without oversight, it's impossible to guarantee what you're actually getting—and that's not a risk I want you to take.

Going Forward Well Informed

Right now, the demand for GLP-1 medications is outpacing drug manufacturers' ability to support it. That's why patient education matters so much. Yes, having an experienced provider is important, but equally as important is your own understanding of how these medications work, what you can expect from them, and how to monitor your progress.

By reading this book, you're equipping yourself with tools and insight that many patients never receive, even from their care team. You've learned how to recognize red flags, ask the right questions, and be an active participant in your treatment. If you're lucky enough to work with a knowledgeable provider, their guidance will be invaluable. But if you're managing much of this on your own, you are still capable of having a safe, successful, and transformative experience.

I know I covered a lot of information, and some of it might not fully click until you have your first injection and start to feel the changes for yourself. In the next chapter, I'll talk about what to expect during your treatment and how to continue to set yourself up for success from dose one.

PART II

Your Life-Changing Journey Begins

CHAPTER 5

Your GLP-1 Journey: What to Expect

Welcome to chapter 5, your personal road map for starting GLP-1 treatment. Whether your first injection is tomorrow, next week, or months away, this chapter will give you a clear picture of what lies ahead. The goal of this chapter isn't just to inform you; it's also to prepare you. When you know what's around the next corner, you can meet each phase of the journey with confidence instead of confusion. You'll be better equipped to recognize progress, troubleshoot any setbacks, and stay engaged. The better you understand the path ahead, the more successful your journey will be.

In the pages ahead, I'll cover all the practicalities of getting started with your treatment: when and how to take your first dose, how your body might feel in the first few days and the first few weeks, and how each dose of the medication works over the course of a week. You'll learn how often to follow up with your doctor, how to recognize what's working (and what's not), and how your relationship with food might change. Just as important, I'll talk about setting realistic expectations. This chapter will guide you through day one *and* beyond; you'll find everything you should know and prepare for in the early days of your GLP-1 journey.

Setting the Right Goals

Before starting treatment, your provider will likely set a weight loss goal with you. However, reaching a certain number on the scale is not the true objective of GLP-1 therapy. **Being skinny is not the goal. Losing fat is the goal. Improving your health meaningfully is the goal.**

It's important to understand that the point of your treatment isn't to decrease your body size or change how your body looks but to promote **body recomposition.** Body recomposition is the process of lowering your overall body fat percentage while preserving (or even building!) muscle mass along the way. Body recomposition gives you a two-for-one deal when it comes to your metabolic health.

Lowering your body fat percentage means that you decrease the amount of visceral fat in your body. This is the dangerous fat around your organs that increases your risk of developing certain diseases. In simple terms, visceral fat is a pro-inflammatory tissue, and it also promotes insulin resistance. Both increase your risk of developing metabolic disorders and cancers such as breast, colon, stomach, and pancreas, to name a few. Increasing your muscle mass, meanwhile, enables you to harness your greatest metabolic asset. As you'll learn in the next chapter, muscle is *essential* for long-term weight maintenance because it is more metabolically active and burns more energy than fat does.

By shifting more of your body composition to the more metabolically active muscle tissue, you will improve your metabolic health, increase your energy level, and make sustainable changes to your long-term health. You can even think of GLP-1 therapy as retraining your metabolism through body recomposition.

While weight loss is often one of the most visible and celebrated outcomes of body recomposition and GLP-1 therapy, I encourage my patients not to rely on the scale as their sole measure of success. Weight is just one data point, and it's often a misleading one. What truly matters is how your body is changing beneath the surface: reduction of visceral fat, preservation or gain of lean muscle mass, improved metabolic markers, and how you feel from day to day.

There may be times when the pace of your weight loss slows or doesn't align with your expectations. That doesn't automatically mean the medication isn't working. It may signal the need for a dosage adjustment, a shift in your nutrition or exercise strategy, or simply more time needed for your body to respond. That's why it's critical to have ongoing, thoughtful conversations with your provider.

By prioritizing body recomposition over weight loss alone, you can stay focused on the bigger goal: building a healthier, stronger, more resilient body, not just a lighter one. That's the real prize.

Why Sustainability Beats Speed

Many patients with overweight and obesity have waited years—sometimes decades—for a tool such as GLP-1 therapy. Once they start, they naturally want to see results as quickly as possible. I completely understand why they might feel impatient. After all, if a low starting dose already has an effect, wouldn't a higher dose get results even faster?

It can be tempting to want the weight gone *yesterday*—but

slow and steady weight loss is more sustainable and healthier in the long run. GLP-1 medications don't kick in overnight, and you wouldn't want them to.

The starting doses of liraglutide, semaglutide, and tirzepatide aren't just arbitrary quantities; they are carefully designed to let your body adapt to the medication and lay the foundation for higher, more effective doses later. Even if you don't see much weight loss at first, these early doses allow you to:

- Experience what being on a GLP-1 feels like
- Notice how your appetite and satiety cues shift
- Learn how your body responds to different foods
- Build the habits that will carry you through maintenance
- Help avoid side effects, such as nausea, vomiting, dehydration, and more (which can sometimes be bad enough to make you want to quit GLP-1 medications altogether if you don't start slow and stay slow)
- Avoid losing weight too quickly and increasing your risk of losing muscle instead of fat

Trying to rush results comes at the cost of sustainability and safety. You're not racing to a finish line; you're building a lifelong relationship with your body and your health.

Recognizing Progress

Since the number of pounds you lose and how fast you lose them won't give you a full picture of whether you're successfully retraining your metabolism, it's important to know what meaningful progress looks like. The signs described in this list reflect real, sustainable changes in your health, even if the scale is moving more slowly than you'd hoped.

- Your body composition analysis shows that you have a lower percentage of body fat and less visceral fat.
- You're maintaining muscle. Ideally, less than 10 percent of your overall weight loss is a result of decreased muscle mass.
- Your cravings are fading. You're experiencing less food noise.
- Your markers for metabolic health are improving. Your blood pressure might be lower, and your blood glucose level might be more stable.
- Your lab results are also improving. Markers such as HbA1c and your lipid panel might improve.
- Your daily life feels easier, even incrementally. You might experience more energy, better sleep, and more comfortable movement.

When taking GLP-1s, small internal shifts often precede significant external changes. If you're expecting fast, dramatic weight loss right out of the gate, you may be discouraged when the scale doesn't move right away, but know that GLP-1s are creating subtle internal shifts before external changes show up. That doesn't mean you're doing anything wrong; progress is happening even if it doesn't seem like it yet. Plus, learning to notice and trust your body's subtle signals will set you up for long-term success. You will not only avoid needlessly worrying about the effectiveness of your medication, but you'll also develop a better understanding of how your body tends to respond to a specific dose. This information will be especially helpful when you need to adjust how much you're taking.

YOU KNOW YOURSELF BEST

When I look at a patient's body composition analysis, I can get a good sense of what weight would likely be ideal for them. But before sharing this number with patients, I first like to ask them at what weight they felt the most comfortable during their adult life. Most of the time, they share a number that is almost exactly what their body composition analysis is telling me—sometimes down to the pound. The fat loss recommended by the body composition analysis nearly always matches the body weight at which the patient felt their best.

I'm amazed each time it happens, and it proves something that I want my patients to understand: You know your body best. When it comes to setting your health goal or at any point in your GLP-1 journey, don't be afraid to speak up about how you're feeling and what you think will work best for you.

How Quickly Will a GLP-1 Start to Work?

You now understand that the initial results of a GLP-1 might not be easy to see at first, but this question might still be at the back of your mind. The answer? It depends; every person responds a little differently, and each medication has its own timeline. Here's what to expect for each GLP-1 drug.

Semaglutide (Wegovy, Ozempic)

> **Starting dose:** You begin at a subtherapeutic dose of 0.25 milligram weekly.
>
> **Titration timeline:** The weekly dose increases by 0.25 milligram at a time, up to a maximum of 2 milligrams for Ozempic or 2.4 milligrams for Wegovy. I usually keep my patients on a 0.25-milligram dose for four weeks, and if they tolerate it, I increase it to 0.5 milligram. From this dose and above, the titration period can vary from patient to patient, but most

doses have an effect within eight to twelve weeks. It's unlikely that I will increase a dose any sooner than this.

When you'll feel it: Some people start feeling the effects of the medication at the 0.25-milligram dose, but most people don't notice any results until their dose hits 0.5 milligram or higher.

Why it's made this way: The slow progression is necessary to minimize nausea and GI-related side effects.

THE LOWEST DOSE STILL MATTERS

The 0.25-milligram dose still plays an important role, even if you don't experience any immediate effects. It will help you tolerate higher doses, where you will see most of the weight loss. Don't be discouraged if the results in the early weeks feel underwhelming—you're still on track.

Tirzepatide (Zepbound, Mounjaro)

Starting dose: You begin at a therapeutic dose of 2.5 milligrams weekly.

Titration timeline: The weekly dose increases by 2.5 milligrams at a time, up to a maximum of 15 milligrams, but some people can stay at lower doses long term. The titration of tirzepatide is different from that of semaglutide, at least with the initial dose. Usually, patients can stay on the first dose of 2.5 milligrams for up to three months and then increase. Remember, the initial dose of 2.5 milligrams of tirzepatide is a therapeutic dose. Some patients can lose up to thirty pounds on the first dose.

When you'll feel it: Many patients report reduced appetite and weight loss as early as the first injections. Some patients may never need to titrate above the 2.5-milligram dose.

Liraglutide (Saxenda, Victoza)

>**Starting dose:** You begin at a subtherapeutic dose of 0.6 milligram daily.
>
>**Titration timeline:** The weekly dose increases by 0.6 milligram at a time, up to a maximum total of 3.0 milligrams. The titration of liraglutide can take place anywhere from eight to twelve weeks after each dose.
>
>**When you'll feel it:** It can take longer to feel an effect from liraglutide, as it's titrated more slowly than other GLP-1 medications due to its more significant side effects.

Subtle Shifts and Early Signs of Progress

Because the effects of GLP-1 medications can be subtle at first, it's easy to second-guess whether they're working or not. This can give you the false idea that you need to increase their dosage in order to see progress. To help manage your expectations, this timeline will give you an overview of the changes that most people taking a GLP-1 see in the early weeks and when to expect them. It will reassure you that progress is often happening—even if it's behind the scenes—and to keep your spirits up if your journey seems stalled before it starts. Remember, your individual timeline will vary depending on your age, medication, and other lifestyle factors. This is just a general look ahead.

>**Weeks 1–2:** You may begin to see appetite changes and a reduction of food noise, especially within the first few days of a dose of tirzepatide. Some patients feel fuller with smaller portions of food. For patients with hypertension, their blood pressure may improve within the first or second week. Some of my patients have reported that they "just feel better"

within the first few days of treatment (which I love to hear!). This feeling of well-being comes too soon to be a result of weight loss, and most often, it's just a direct result of having less pro-inflammatory food in your system. Other patients feel little or no effect at this stage, especially if they're on semaglutide. Again, this is not a sign of failure; it's how the medication initially works. Don't forget: Internal changes often begin before external ones do.

Weeks 3–6: If you're on tirzepatide or have titrated to a higher dose of semaglutide, this is often when the appetite suppression really kicks in. Many patients describe a dramatic reduction in food noise at this point.

Weeks 6–12: This is when many patients start to notice changes, both in how they feel and with their weight. Now might be the time to increase your dose. A good way to know is if the appetite suppression effect starts to wear off prior to your next injection. If you're starting to think, "Maybe I should do my shot earlier," pause. The solution to this problem isn't to inject the medication more often; it's to contact your provider and ask about increasing your dose. During this time, many patients reach the point where they feel more comfortable—both physically and mentally—to start exercising again, which is another important milestone. You may begin to feel more comfortable with increasing your protein intake and strength training (I'll discuss how these two practices fit into your treatment in chapter 6).

The bottom line? Don't try to judge progress too early, and don't try to compare your timeline to anyone else's, especially if someone at home or close to you is also taking these medications. I have two sets of identical twins as patients, and *each twin* responds differently.

Navigating Changes in Hunger Cues and Food Consumption

One of the most profound changes you'll experience on GLP-1 medications is the way you relate to food: how you think about it, how much you want it, and how it makes you feel. The shifts go beyond simply feeling full sooner. Your body's reward pathways are being rewired, helping to quiet cravings and reduce the constant mental chatter about food. These changes can feel surprising, even unsettling, at first, so here's what you can expect as your relationship with food evolves.

Rewiring Your Relationship with Food

Remember, GLP-1 receptor agonists don't just act on the stomach, they also work in the brain, particularly in the areas that regulate appetite, satiety, and the reward system. They reduce the drive to eat and seek out hyperpalatable foods. These foods are designed with specific combinations of fat, salt, sugar, and carbohydrates that light up your brain's dopamine pathways and create cravings, compulsions, and food noise. (Examples include sugar-filled snacks, processed carbs, and fast food.)

With GLP-1s, the chatter about food is turned down—drastically. You feel fuller after eating half of what you would normally need to feel full. You enjoy your food while eating, but you become physically satisfied with smaller portions.

For many people, GLP-1 medications relieve a huge emotional and cognitive burden. You won't think about whether you should snack in between meals. You may find that the things you used to crave no longer hold the same appeal. You might take a few bites and find yourself uninterested in finishing the full portion. You'll find that the constant mental gymnastics about what, when, and how much to eat start to fade away.

GARY'S STORY

I had struggled with my weight my entire life, seesawing with large swings as I tried various methods over the years. Through it all, the food noise in my head never went away. I obsessed about food, my weight, and my appearance—no matter what I had eaten or what the scale said.

As covid came to an end and my wife gave birth to our second child, I woke up realizing that I was at my heaviest ever—and miserable when I should have been incredibly happy. Upon a friend's recommendation, I started semaglutide. Within a year, I had lost eighty pounds. Even more significant was the mental relief. The constant obsession with food lifted, and for the first time, I wasn't thinking about food all day.

Since then, I've stayed on a low-maintenance dose, and my weight has remained stable. I've never been happier with my body or my life.

A New Kind of Satisfaction

When starting GLP-1 therapy, many of my patients ask me, "Will I still enjoy food?" This is a very common—and valid—concern that many patients beginning their medication have. The short answer to this question is "yes." GLP-1s don't take away your ability to enjoy food, but what enjoyment of food looks like and the role food plays in your life might look different. You'll still find pleasure in a meal, but you might notice that you no longer need to clean your plate to feel satisfied or that indulgent foods don't trigger the same emotional response they used to. If you've spent years using food for comfort, distraction, reward, or stress relief, this shift can feel particularly profound. GLP-1 medications can help you decouple those associations, giving you the chance to build new habits and undo the patterns that lead to emotional eating.

Still, some patients are concerned that if they no longer find food rewarding, life might feel . . . flat. Food plays many roles in our lives. It helps celebrate holidays, sparks memories, and can commemorate milestones. Losing the rush of a sugar high or the joy of a favorite treat can feel disorienting at first, especially if food has been one of your primary sources of pleasure throughout your life. But what many patients find is that this initial discomfort is short-lived. In its place? *Peace.* A sense of control. Freedom from the tug-of-war between desire and guilt.

Many patients on GLP-1 therapy discover new sources of joy and connection. Not only do they feel physically better but they are able to show up fully in social settings or finally have the energy to try new activities. In short, you don't lose the pleasure you experienced before starting a GLP-1; it just appears in other parts of your life.

This shift away from food as a primary source of comfort or control often feels like liberation. For the first time, patients find that they're not spending all day negotiating with themselves, their cravings, or their guilt about eating certain foods; this mental space is freed up. They can finally glimpse the life ahead of them—one that's fueled by food but not ruled by it.

GLP-1s and Alcohol

Many patients are surprised by how their relationship with alcohol changes when they are on a GLP-1. Much the same way as these medications quiet "food noise," they seem to turn down the volume on alcohol cravings—often without any conscious effort on your part.

Remember how GLP-1 agonists act on the brain, especially the areas responsible for reward, motivation, and compulsion? Alcohol, like hyperpalatable food, taps into these circuits. It activates dopamine pathways that create a feeling of pleasure, comfort, and escape. If you've ever reached for a glass of wine to unwind at the end of the day or relied on a cocktail to ease into a social setting, you've already experienced how those associations can become reflexive.

But GLP-1s disrupt that loop. What once felt rewarding may now feel muted. That familiar glass of wine after work might not bring the same sense of relief. A drink at a party might lose its appeal halfway through. And for many patients, the internal urge—the automatic pull toward alcohol—simply goes away. This isn't just an anecdotal effect; GLP-1 agonists are being studied as potential treatments for alcohol dependency.

This doesn't mean that you can't drink while on a GLP-1. For most people, it's generally safe to consume alcohol in moderation, and some patients continue to enjoy it without issue. But it does mean that your experience of drinking may change. You might notice that you're feeling a little more sensitive to it; it takes less alcohol to start feeling a buzz. But the more notable change is that you may no longer feel the same emotional return on investment: the habit is still there, but the reward has shifted.

You may still enjoy a glass of wine or choose to toast at a wedding. But you may also find that you don't need the drink to feel relaxed, fun, or connected. Like food, alcohol is woven into our social lives, celebrations, and memories, and it can feel strange when something that once marked a special occasion no longer delivers the same effect. But similar to what happens with food, what often replaces the buzz is a sense of clarity and control.

An Opportunity for Change

Once GLP-1s start to quiet your cravings and loosen the grip of emotional eating, one of the most powerful (and underrated) effects of the medication emerges: a new level of awareness. That awareness gives you the opportunity to observe your habits—and begin reshaping them. The earlier you begin to take advantage of this opportunity, the more confident and prepared you'll be for long-term success.

GLP-1s make your old, automatic patterns (such as cleaning your plate, reaching for something sweet after a stressful moment, or snacking out of boredom) easier to identify and interrupt. They help reduce the emotional charge behind cravings and create a buffer between the impulse and the action. The effects of GLP-1s not only reshape past behaviors around food; you may also notice that they help you to start new habits. The medication makes it easier to focus, decide, and follow through on the changes you want to make.

That makes this the perfect time to start practicing the habits that will carry you forward. With the medication helping to quiet the noise from cravings and emotion-driven eating, you may find it easier to focus, follow through, and build new routines. These aren't dramatic changes but simple shifts that you can start now—ones that will support you throughout your treatment. They'll also help you feel more prepared if you decide to lower your dose for maintenance or go off the medication later.

- **Plan your meals and snacks ahead of time.** With your hunger cues changing, you may find yourself spending extended periods of time without eating, and as a result, you won't have enough time in your day to consume the necessary amount of protein to maximize fat loss and minimize muscle loss. Eating at regular intervals helps you consume enough protein and maintain consistent energy throughout the day.
- **Think about the structure of your meals.** Spoiler alert: You'll learn much more about this in chapter 6. For now,

just know that it'll be important for you to prioritize certain nutrients over others—but not in a restrictive way or as a "diet."
- Focus on your experience of eating. When eating, try to notice how food tastes, how it feels in your body, and when you start feeling satisfied. These cues and patterns will get stronger the more you pay attention to them.

You won't always feel this clear and focused. Life will get noisy again. But at this stage of your journey, the medication should be doing a lot of heavy lifting for you, so that makes this the perfect moment to build the foundation. If you build new habits that will help you approach food differently, they'll be there for you later when you want to lower your dose or eventually stop treatment altogether. You don't have to overhaul your life with new habits all at once, but if you start small and stay consistent, this can be the moment where everything starts to shift.

EATING OUT

You may notice that dining out while on a GLP-1 feels different than it used to. Your appetite is lower, the portions seem enormous, and meals can feel overwhelming instead of enjoyable. What I often recommend in this situation is simple:
- Consider ordering an appetizer as your main dish.
- Split an entree with a friend.
- If dining alone, plan to take half your meal home for the next day.

Your capacity is different now, but think of it as an opportunity to slow down and be more intentional about what foods you really enjoy.

Practical Tips for a Smooth Start

Let's shift our focus to something a little more practical: the logistics of taking your medication. From choosing your start day to storing your prescription properly, considering a few key details can make a big difference.

Choosing Your Start Day

One practical decision that patients sometimes don't often consider is deciding which day of the week to take their injection. I typically recommend starting on a Friday, and here's why:

- **Appetite suppression peaks when you need it most.** Weekends tend to bring more social events, indulgent meals, and alcohol. GLP-1s are most effective in reducing appetite during the first few days after your injection, so starting on a Friday means that you'll have the support of the medication when you're most likely to need it.
- **You'll be able to manage potential side effects more easily.** Common side effects such as nausea, fatigue, or GI discomfort are more manageable at home. If you start on a Friday, you'll have the weekend to rest and monitor your body's response without needing to miss work or school (staying home isn't as fun as it may seem when you're feeling unwell).
- **You'll avoid the "expiration effect" falling on the weekend.** After several weeks on the same dose, some patients notice that the effects of the medication begin to wear off earlier—sometimes as soon as day five instead of day seven. If you inject on a Monday, that drop-off will happen on a Friday or Saturday—again, when cravings or overeating tendencies might be strongest. Starting on a Friday shifts that window to midweek, helping you stay more consistent with your weight loss.

That said, not every patient's life follows this pattern. If your weekends are quiet and your weekdays are busier, another start day might work better for you and your lifestyle. The key is to understand your lifestyle and plan accordingly.

CHANGING YOUR INJECTION DAY

If your schedule changes and you need to switch your injection day, you can do so. I recommend that patients move their injection back one day a time per week. Here's an example: If your injection day is Sunday and you would rather do it on Thursday, I would recommend doing the injection on Saturday of the first week; the second week, do the injection on Friday; and the third week, do it on Thursday and stay there.

Mastering Injections

Many patients have never had to inject themselves with medication, and it can feel a little intimidating. But with the right technique, it quickly becomes second nature. (I have patients as young as twelve years old who can inject by themselves.) Whether you're using a self-injecting pen or a syringe, here are some best practices to ensure comfort, safety, and effectiveness from day one.

- **Rotate injection sites weekly.** To avoid irritation, use different areas of your body each week; the abdomen, thighs, and upper arms are the most common areas. For semaglutide pen injections, pinch an inch of fat at the site before injecting. This helps the medication get into your subcutaneous fat, which is where it absorbs best.
- **Know how to treat irritation at the injection site.** Redness, itching, or a mild, localized rash can be common, especially with Zepbound, and is generally nothing to worry too much about. If you experience this, I usually recommend applying a thin film of hydrocortisone cream

to the affected area before the next shot. If you frequently experience a lot of itchiness, you can take Zyrtec the day of the injection. However, if you experience swelling beyond the injection area, hives, difficulty breathing, or a rapid heartbeat, you need to seek medical attention immediately.

Storing and Transporting Your Medication

Keeping your medication at the right temperature is essential to maintaining its potency and safety. Here's what you need to know about storage, both at home and outside.

- **Refrigeration is key.** Before their first use, GLP-1 medications should always be stored in the refrigerator between 36 and 46 degrees Fahrenheit. Once open, some medications can stay at room temperature for longer periods of time, but others must always be kept in the refrigerator. Check the storage instructions for your specific medication.
- **Refrigerate, never freeze, the medication.** If your medication accidentally freezes, it's no longer safe or effective and should be discarded. Make sure your refrigerator doesn't have any extra-cold spots.
- **Travel with a cooler.** If you're going on a trip and need to take your medication with you, pack your pen in a travel cooler with an ice pack. If you are flying, keep it in your carry-on in case of lost checked luggage for a short flight, but for a long direct flight, you may want to consider putting it into your checked luggage because of the cold temperature in the cargo hold. You should also make sure that your medication is clearly labeled, ideally in its original packaging with the prescription label, to avoid any issues with airport security.

Going to Your Follow-up Appointments

Follow-up visits are an important part of staying on track with your treatment. These check-ins give you and your provider the chance to evaluate how things have been going, whether your dosage needs to be adjusted, and whether you're getting the results you hoped for. If you've had any side effects or questions about how you've been feeling, this is the time to talk about them.

I typically like to see my patients for a follow-up about six to eight weeks after their initial visit. (Depending on your provider and treatment plan, you might have a longer stretch of time between appointments, closer to eight to twelve weeks.) That's usually enough time to assess how they are tolerating the medication, what's happening with their appetite, and—critically—what's happening with their body composition. At this visit, we repeat their body composition analysis and review their experience so far. They have the opportunity to go over every question they have had since starting treatment. This is also the moment when everything starts to click for the patient.

Until you've been on one of these medications, it's hard to fully understand the changes they'll bring. For many people, it almost sounds like science fiction—too good to be true. That's why I love the first follow-up visit; now we're finally speaking the same language.

Before each appointment, it really helps to prepare; you'll find a checklist for follow-up appointments in the back of the book. Many patients find that they forget what they want to ask once they're in the doctor's room. Taking a moment with the follow-up appointment checklist—or better yet, taking it with you to your appointment—will help you get the most out of the one-on-one time with your doctor.

Monitoring Progress with Body Composition

I always like to remind my patients and my followers that GLP-1 agonists are sophisticated medications that require sophisticated measurements. The most sophisticated measurements? They come from body composition analysis.

As mentioned in the earlier chapters, one of the most important tools in your journey will be your body composition analysis. I spoke about body composition analysis in the context of diagnosing obesity back in chapter 1, but it's not just for screening potential candidates for GLP-1 therapy; it's also the best way to track your results over time and ensure that you are losing fat without losing muscle. Your provider will also use body composition scans to determine whether to adjust your GLP-1 dose. The most common scans that providers use to assess body composition include:

- **Magnetic resonance imaging (MRI) scan:** The gold standard for measuring visceral fat, but because it's expensive to have done frequently and cumbersome, it is not widely used for routine assessments.

- **Dual-energy X-ray absorptiometry (DEXA) scan:** The second-best option for measuring visceral fat, DEXA machines use low-level X-rays to differentiate among bone, fat, and lean tissue. They provide accurate measurements of body fat, muscle mass, and bone density, but like MRIs, they are not commonly used for frequent body composition reports.

- **Body impedance analysis (BIA):** This is a method of estimating body composition by measuring how electrical currents move through the body. Since muscle, fat, and water conduct electricity differently, this technique helps determine the proportions of lean mass, fat mass, and total body water. While not as precise as an MRI or a DEXA scan, a BIA is a practical and accessible tool for tracking changes in body composition over time—especially during weight loss. It shifts the focus away from the number on the scale and provides a more meaningful look at what's actually changing inside your body. This is what I use to track changes in body composition in my office.

What Body Composition Scans Can Tell Us

At every follow-up visit, I perform a body composition analysis, and if your provider offers this at their practice, I recommend you follow the same cadence. Here's what I look at every time I review a patient's body composition report:

- **Skeletal muscle mass** (how much of your body is skeletal muscle, the muscle you can build with strength training)
- **Percentage body fat** (how much of your body is fat tissue)
- **Visceral fat** (how much dangerous fat is stored around your organs)

Muscle-Fat Analysis

		55	70	85	100	115	130	145	160	175	190	205 %
Weight	(lb)							157.1				
Skeletal Muscle Mass (SMM)	(lb)	70	80	90	100	110	120	130	140	150	160	170 %
						51.8						
Body Fat Mass	(lb)	40	60	80	100	160	220	280	340	400	460	520 %
									64.3			

This is a suboptimal body composition. The report shows more body fat than skeletal muscle mass (SMM). If we connect the ends of the three bars, they make a letter C.

Muscle-Fat Analysis

		55	70	85	100	115	130	145	160	175	190	205 %
Weight	(lb)				113.2							
Skeletal Muscle Mass (SMM)	(lb)	70	80	90	100	110	120	130	140	150	160	170 %
					49.4							
Body Fat Mass	(lb)	40	60	80	100	160	220	280	340	400	460	520 %
					24.4							

This report is from the same patient four years later. Their body composition is now optimal. The bars in the report form a letter D.

Muscle-Fat Analysis

		55	70	85	100	115	130	145	160	175	190	205 %
Weight	(lb)								216.5			
Skeletal Muscle Mass (SMM)	(lb)	70	80	90	100	110	120	130	140	150	160	170 %
								73.9				
Body Fat Mass	(lb)	40	60	80	100	160	220	280	340	400	460	520 %
										83.6		

This is another suboptimal "C-shaped" body composition. You can see that this patient has plenty of skeletal muscle mass, but their body fat mass is still high relative to their skeletal muscle mass.

Muscle-Fat Analysis

		55	70	85	100	115	130	145	160	175	190	205 %
Weight	(lb)						171.2					
Skeletal Muscle Mass (SMM)	(lb)	70	80	90	100	110	120	130	140	150	160	170 %
							69.9					
Body Fat Mass	(lb)	40	60	80	100	160	220	280	340	400	460	520 %
							44.2					

This is the same patient two years later, with a corrected proportion of muscle mass to body fat. This is a great example of body recomposition!

Other helpful information that your body composition report can share includes:

- **Where you tend to store fat:** If you store more fat in your trunk and upper extremities, you're at greatest risk of having high visceral fat, metabolic syndrome, insulin resistance, and type 2 diabetes. If you store more fat in your hips and thighs, you may have a greater risk of cardiovascular disease. Understanding fat distribution helps us identify the types of metabolic risk you may face and how aggressively we need to intervene.
- **Muscle mass by body segment (arms, legs, trunk):** This breakdown helps determine if muscle loss is occurring uniformly or in specific areas. It's not just the total muscle mass that matters, but how it's distributed, especially when evaluating changes over time.
- **Target recommendations for fat loss and muscle gain based on your unique body composition:** These are tailored estimates based on your measurements, showing how much fat you may need to lose and how much muscle you could benefit from building. These targets help us personalize your plan and track your progress.

Based on my experience reviewing thousands of body composition reports, a healthy pace for fat loss that doesn't sacrifice significant muscle mass is anywhere from 0.5 to 1 pound of fat per week. We'll discuss why losing fat without losing muscle is considered metabolic success in the next chapter.

How to Monitor Body Composition at Home

Ideally, every follow-up visit with your doctor should include a body composition scan. I say ideally because the reality is that many doctors' offices and telehealth providers still don't invest in this technology. If your doctor doesn't offer body composition scans, you can invest in an at-home body composition scale. A regular bathroom scale will not give you an idea of whether the weight you're losing is fat, muscle, or a combination of the two. But if it's not economically feasible for you to purchase one for home use, you may want to check to see if one is available at a gym near you. If not, don't worry; I'll also show you other ways to track your progress in "Tracking Progress Without a Body Composition Scale" on page 125.

I ask patients to assess changes about every two to three weeks at home if they have access to a BIA machine or a smart scale using these tips for getting the most accurate measurements.

- **Choose a scale with the right features.** The scales with the most accurate readings use multifrequency bioelectrical impedance analysis (BIA), both foot and hand electrodes, and segmental analysis to assess fat and muscle distribution in various body parts, including the torso.
- **Take your measurements under similar conditions.** Aim to do so at the same time of day (first thing in the morning is best), before eating or drinking and after going to the bathroom.
- **Focus on overall trends, not day-to-day numbers.** Small fluctuations are normal; what matters is the bigger picture over weeks, not small ups and downs. I recommend taking a measurement at home no more than once every two weeks.
- **Know that hydration will affect your results.** Try not to be dehydrated or overhydrated when you take your measurements, as being either will skew your body fat reading.
- **Avoid measuring right after intense exercise.** A strenuous workout temporarily changes your body's fluid balance and can distort your results.

TRACKING PROGRESS WITHOUT A BODY COMPOSITION SCALE

While I strongly encourage you to invest in a home body composition scale if possible, I understand that it's not always an option. If you're not able to monitor your body composition closely:

- **Track your protein intake.** You'll learn the importance of tracking your protein intake in the next chapter, but keeping tabs on your protein intake is essential for people who are not able to keep a close eye on their muscle loss and development. It'll be crucial for you to hit your daily protein minimum, so you may want to keep a journal to track what you're eating to make sure you're not overestimating your protein intake and follow the guidelines for protein consumption in the next chapter.
- **Pay attention to how you feel.** If you're feeling stronger and more energetic as you move through your everyday life, that's a powerful sign of fat loss and improved health.
- **Notice how your clothes fit.** Often, patients notice that they've dropped a pants size or find that their clothes fit more loosely, even if the number on the scale hasn't changed dramatically.

What Comes Next: The Building Blocks of Lasting Change

Starting your medication is a huge step on your GLP-1 journey. So . . . is that it? Can you just inject yourself and watch the fat loss commence? No! As I'm sure you're beginning to grasp by now, starting GLP-1 therapy isn't as simple as just taking a medication.

In the next chapter, we'll get strategic. We'll dive into the two major lifestyle factors that will define your muscle retention and long-term success: protein consumption and strength training. I know that "lifestyle change" can feel like a loaded term, especially if you've been through diets and plans that never delivered on their promises. The difference is that this time, you also have a medication that actually works. You'll learn how to maximize your results—and keep them for good.

CHAPTER 6

Staying on Course: Your GPS for Progress

By this point in your journey, you've learned a lot about GLP-1 medications. You understand how they work, why they were developed, and what makes them such a powerful tool in the treatment of overweight and obesity. You've laid a solid foundation. I hear you, I see you, and I am so happy for you. Now we'll walk the rest of the path together.

While GLP-1s are an important part of your treatment, they're just one part. To get the best results—and, more important, to keep them—you need a full plan. That means pairing your medication with two other essential components: the right nutrition and the right type of movement.

In this chapter, you'll learn what it takes to get the most out of your GLP-1 treatment—and how to set yourself up for long-term success. GLP-1s are powerful targeted medications developed to work in complex, elegant ways inside your body. To get the most out of them—in terms of both results and how you feel—you need more than just a prescription; you need to know what's going on behind the scenes. Your doctor may not have the time or knowledge to walk you through this level of detail, but that doesn't mean you don't deserve to have it.

This is where lifestyle changes come into play. If you already have healthy habits in place, such as regular exercise or a higher-protein diet, this part of the journey may be easy. If not, don't worry. You're not expected to figure out everything right away. We'll take baby steps together.

Contrary to popular belief, choosing GLP-1 treatment isn't the "easy way out." There's real work ahead—maybe the kind you've never done before. The effort you put into your lifestyle regarding physical activity and nutrition will determine your early and long-term success. But here's the great news: If you do the work, this time it will actually pay off.

You've made an informed, proactive decision to take care of your health—and there's nothing shameful about that. If some part of you feels as though you're supposed to suffer to "deserve" progress, it's time to unlearn that. With the right support, strategy, and structure, the effort you put in now will translate into whole-body health that you can feel and see—and *keep*.

Introducing the GPS: Guiding You to Optimal Results

Whenever you navigate unfamiliar territory, it helps to have a system that will keep you on course. When you're lost, you ask for directions. You'll use the same principle here. You have a secret weapon for success in your GLP-1 journey: I call it your GPS. In this book, GPS has a different meaning from what you're used to:

G stands for GLP-1

P stands for Protein, and

S stands for Strength training

Easy enough to remember, right? This GPS system is a clear, flexible road map for your treatment plan. While you've already spent a lot of time learning about GLP-1 medications, this chapter is where we'll turn our attention to the two other crucial factors. You'll learn what to eat and how to move to best support your body. I like to call the GPS the "three prescriptions of treatment"; each is an equally essential piece of the puzzle.

G Is for GLP-1

You have learned a lot about GLP-1s by now. You know how they help regulate appetite and improve metabolic health, but there is another crucial lesson to learn: **Your long-term success on GLP-1s will depend on your maintaining muscle-preserving habits.** GLP-1s must work *with* these habits; they don't work *in place of* them.

Before I break down the P and the S of your GPS, let's pause to see why muscle matters so much. Once you know the role muscle plays—not just in how your body looks but also in how it functions—you'll never think about weight loss the same way again.

Muscle Matters

What is muscle, and why is it one of your body's most valuable assets? The human body contains three types of muscles:

1. **Cardiac muscle,** which makes up the heart and pumps blood through your circulatory system.

2. **Smooth muscle,** which lines your blood vessels and organs and works to keep things such as your digestion and circulation going. This activity is involuntary, meaning that you don't control it.

3. **Skeletal muscle** is what people usually think of when they hear the word *muscle;* it's the kind you can flex, strengthen, and, more important, *build.* It's also the kind we'll be focusing on here.

Most of us think of skeletal muscle as something that helps with strength and mobility, and those are very important functions. But it does so much more than that. It is a metabolically active, **endocrine-responsive tissue.**

Whenever skeletal muscle contracts (no matter if you're lifting weights, climbing stairs, or just going about your day), it releases **myokines.** These chemical messengers travel through your bloodstream and help coordinate some key functions across your body. Myokines have positive effects on metabolic, cardiovascular, mental, and immunological processes. They help your liver manage glucose, improve your insulin sensitivity, help your body utilize fat tissue for energy, and even support the health of your pancreas and brain. Every time muscle contracts, it protects your body from being in a chronic inflammatory state. It protects you from disease. It even helps stabilize your mood and cognitive function.

Muscle is metabolically active and highly adaptable, especially during movement. At rest, it burns more calories than fat tissue does (though less per gram than organs such as the brain and liver do).

But during physical activity, muscle is your body's primary energy consumer. Resistance and endurance exercises dramatically increase the amount of energy your muscles demand. The more muscle mass you have, the greater your capacity to burn calories—not just during a workout but for hours after.

Put simply: Muscle burns fat to move. The more muscle you have, the more energy your body needs, which means you burn more fat to meet that need. The more muscle mass you have, the more energy your body needs and the more fat you burn to provide that energy. Isn't the body amazing?

Muscle, GLP-1s, and Defense Against Cancer

We've already talked about how muscle helps regulate inflammation and immunity—but what's becoming increasingly clear is that these same mechanisms may play a role in defense against cancer. While this is still an emerging field, researchers are starting to connect the dots among muscle mass, metabolic health, and cancer outcomes. Several important reasons are that muscle improves insulin sensitivity, reducing chronic hyperinsulinemia (a state that can fuel cancer growth). The release of myokines has an anti-inflammatory effect; they regulate glucose in the bloodstream, providing less energy to cancer cells to multiply. It also provides a buffer during cancer treatment, helping patients tolerate chemotherapy and recover more effectively.

GLP-1 medications may also strengthen this defense system by complementing muscle's metabolic benefits with their own effects on insulin regulation, inflammation, and visceral fat, each of which contributes to making a less hospitable environment for cancer cells to thrive in. Early studies even suggest that GLP-1s may interfere with the way some cancer cells process glucose, although this remains a developing area of research.

> None of this means that GLP-1s are cancer treatments or prevention plans. But together, muscle mass and GLP-1 medications appear to interrupt several of the metabolic and inflammatory pathways that support tumor growth, especially in people with obesity or insulin resistance. These added benefits reflect a deeper truth: While the goal of GLP-1 treatment may be fat loss and improved metabolic health, what you're building is a stronger foundation for your overall long-term wellness.

Most people have no idea how important muscle is until they start losing it. Unfortunately, that's exactly what can happen with GLP-1 treatment if you don't eat enough protein or challenge your muscles.

Muscle loss is often blamed on GLP-1 medications, but it's not the medication itself that is damaging your muscles. Any rapid weight loss, no matter how it happens, will affect your muscle mass. But it's even more crucial to preserve muscle when you are on a GLP-1 because you will eat less while taking the medication. And when you eat less (especially without prioritizing the nutrients your muscles need), your body will pull muscle from its reserves. Muscle is easy for your body to break down. If you're not feeding it and challenging it, your body sees it as expendable. Lose too much, and you'll slow your metabolism, reduce your functional strength, and even increase your risk of future disease. I promise you, blindly losing weight without protecting your muscles will leave you feeling anything but strong. This is why in the last chapter I emphasized that your goal isn't just to make a number on the scale go down; it is to lose fat—*without losing muscle.*

With the right guidance, you can preserve and even *build* skeletal muscle while losing fat. And if you protect your muscles, you'll set yourself up for fat loss that's more efficient and longer-lasting. How?

- **Your first priority is keeping the muscles you have.** That's what protein is for.
- **Your second priority is challenging your muscles just enough to keep them strong**—and hopefully make them grow! That's what strength training is for.

Achieving these priorities won't happen by accident, and that's what the rest of this chapter is about.

P Is for Protein

If skeletal muscle is the engine that powers your body's metabolism, protein is the fuel. It's what enables your body to build, preserve, and repair lean muscle mass—and it's a nonnegotiable priority during GLP-1 treatment.

You may be noticing more and more talk about protein lately; it may seem like the latest fad that everyone is talking about. I usually tell patients to ignore fad diets. But you need to pay attention to your protein intake. While protein consumption definitely seems to be having a moment, it is far from a passing trend. We've known that protein is one of the most important macronutrients for a very long time. Protein builds and preserves muscle, but it goes far beyond that; it is also important for the production of collagen, elastin, bone mass, and satiety, among many other functions.

Protein is especially crucial when you're on a GLP-1 because it provides essential nourishment for your skeletal muscle. To maintain muscle mass, you must give it adequate protein. To stimulate growth, you will require even more. Protein has the highest thermic effect of any macronutrient; your body uses 20 to 30 percent of the calories from protein just to digest and process it. This extra energy demand not only raises your metabolic rate but can also push your body toward greater fat oxidation, meaning that you will burn more fat for fuel. In other words, it helps your body stay in fat-burning mode.

How Much Protein Do You Need?

The dietary guidelines for protein consumption differ depending on who you ask. The United States Department of Agriculture (USDA) recommends 0.8 gram of protein per kilogram of body weight per day. This is about 0.36 gram per pound, so for a 150-pound person, the recommendation would be 54 grams of protein per day. Here's the catch: Most official guidelines are designed to prevent deficiency, not to promote optimal health. These guidelines won't help you preserve or build muscle to thrive as you age.

Many experts, including myself, now recommend **1.2 to 2.0 grams per kilogram of body weight per day** for active individuals, older adults, and those trying to lose weight or preserve muscle. That's about **80 to 135 grams per day** for someone weighing 150 pounds. These targets are backed by organizations such as the International Society of Sports Nutrition (ISSN) and the European Society for Clinical Nutrition and Metabolism (ESPEN). They are published in journals such as *The American Journal of Clinical Nutrition*.

In clinical practice, I've found that a minimum of 100 grams per day is typically necessary just to hold on to existing muscle mass during GLP-1 treatment. And 100 grams per day is a goal that is within your reach, even when you are on a GLP-1.

Complete Proteins

Are all dietary proteins created equal? The short answer is no. Let me explain.

I've talked about the importance of preserving skeletal muscle mass, and I've covered how much protein you need to do that. But choosing the right protein matters; not all proteins will preserve—or grow—muscle tissue. For that to happen, the protein you eat must be a complete protein.

What makes a protein complete? It comes down to amino acids, the building blocks of protein. Just as letters make up words, amino acids make up proteins, which your body uses for nearly everything: hormone production, enzyme function, immune regulation, tissue repair, and more. There are twenty amino acids used by the human body, and they fall into two categories: essential and nonessential.

ESSENTIAL AMINO ACIDS	NONESSENTIAL AMINO ACIDS
Histidine	Alanine
Isoleucine	Arginine
Leucine	Asparagine
Lysine	Aspartic acid
Methionine	(aspartate)
Phenylalanine	Cysteine
Threonine	Glutamic acid
Tryptophan	(glutamate)
Valine	Glutamine
	Glycine
	Proline
	Serine
	Tyrosine

Your body can synthesize nonessential proteins from other nutrients and make them on its own, assuming that you're getting adequate nutrition. It can't, however, create essential amino acids; you must get them from food. To preserve or build muscle, you need to regularly eat protein sources that contain all nine of them. Many sources of complete protein are **animal based**. They include:

- Eggs
- Whey protein
- Casein
- Meat (steak, ground beef, etc.)
- Pork
- Lamb
- Venison
- Poultry (chicken, turkey, duck)
- Fish and seafood (salmon, tuna, sardines, etc.)
- Dairy products (milk, yogurt, cottage cheese)

WHEY PROTEIN AND LEUCINE

Whey protein is considered a complete protein and contains the twenty amino acids that are important for muscle protein synthesis. Whey protein also has the highest leucine content of any complete protein source (about 2.5 grams of protein per 25-gram serving). Why is this important? Because leucine is the key amino acid that activates the pathway that drives muscle protein synthesis. And because it's digested quickly, it's the ideal post-workout supplement when your muscles are most primed for repair and growth.

What about plant-based complete proteins? It's possible—though not necessarily recommended—to meet the protein goals a GLP-1 requires while on a plant-based diet, but you'll need to be even more strategic. If you rely heavily on plant proteins, it's best to combine complementary incomplete proteins (for example, rice and beans or hummus with whole-wheat pita) to help round out the amino acid profile of your meals. For those who follow a vegetarian diet, adding whey protein is one of the easiest ways to make sure your muscle is getting everything it needs (see the box on page 136 to learn more).

Some examples of **plant-based complete proteins** are:
- Soy (tofu, tempeh, edamame)
- Quinoa
- Buckwheat
- Amaranth
- Chia seeds (slightly low in lysine but still considered a nearly complete protein)
- Hemp seeds
- Spirulina (technically an alga)

Most plant-based proteins are missing one or more essential amino acids, but by pairing the right foods, you can create complete proteins. You don't need to eat them at the same meal; as long as you combine complementary protein sources over the course of the day, your body can still get all the essential amino acids it needs. Here are some simple combinations that do just that:
- Lentils + rice
- Beans + grains
- Hummus (or falafel) + pita
- Whole-wheat bread + peanut butter
- Corn tortillas + black beans
- Tahini + chickpeas

Guidelines for Hitting Your Protein Goals

Reaching these protein goals is an adjustment for most people; it's a lot more than they are used to eating, even if they aren't on a GLP-1! Eating this much more protein takes some thought. When you're taking a medication that suppresses your appetite, meeting your daily protein requirement may feel like mission impossible. But it is not hopeless; my patients do it all the time.

Increasing your protein intake isn't just about knowing what to eat; it's about when, how often, and in what form. Logistics, not motivation, tend to be the biggest stumbling block. To help you manage these, here is a protein game plan with six simple guidelines to follow:

1. **Aim to consume 100+ grams of protein per day.** To preserve muscle while losing weight, you need enough total protein if you're on a GLP-1. That means at least 100 grams a day—minimum!

2. **Start early.** Getting a solid dose of protein within the first hour or so of waking up gives you a head start and helps distribute your intake across the day, which is much easier on your appetite than trying to cram it all in at the end. If you're someone who puts creamer or milk into your coffee, add a scoop of unflavored or flavored whey protein instead.

3. **Count no more than 30 grams of protein per meal.** I once had a patient who was using two servings of protein powder at a time. Double the serving, double the protein, right? Unfortunately, no. He may have been consuming twice the recommended amount, but his body was utilizing only half of it. Research shows that 30 grams is about the maximum amount of protein your body will direct toward muscle

preservation/development at any given meal. Aim to space your daily protein intake across four portions, each with around 25 to 30 grams of protein at a time. (Don't know what 30 grams of protein looks like? Turn to the Protein Cheat Sheet on page 228 for a quick guide.) If your meal goes over 30 grams of protein, that's fine—but make sure you're only counting the 30 grams that your body actually processed toward your daily total.

4. **Give your body time between meals.** Space your meals at least three to four hours apart. Protein is very filling; if you don't allow enough time between supplementation and meals, you won't be able to consume the amount of protein you need in a day.

5. **Get the protein off your plate first.** This will ensure that you meet your target protein intake even if your appetite dips midway through your meal.

6. **Drink protein shakes.** Protein shakes and powders are a great way to supplement (more on choosing a good one below). Many patients are successful with keeping to a roughly fifty/fifty ratio of protein shakes to meals. This ensures that you have a quick and easy way to load up on protein but don't end up feeling undernourished or experiencing low energy from lack of food. As you plan your day, remember not to have any shakes too close to meals; you don't want a shake making you feel full when it's time to eat!

You can also find these guidelines in the Protein Cheat Sheet on page 228 for quick reference throughout your GLP-1 journey.

CHOOSING A PROTEIN POWDER

There are thousands of protein powders out there—but don't let the endless labels and flavors overwhelm you. The right one for you is the one you'll actually use and that supports your goals without a lot of extra ingredients your body doesn't need. Here's what to look for:

- **Keep it simple.** Choose a product with as few ingredients as possible. Ideally, your protein powder should have one main ingredient, such as grass-fed whey isolate or concentrate, and maybe a few others (such as cacao or stevia) if it's flavored or sweetened. Skip anything with long lists of additives, gums, or sugar alcohols if you're sensitive to them.

- **Prioritize complete proteins.** If you're not eating a fully plant-based diet, a whey protein isolate is usually the most effective option for a complete protein; it's highly digestible and is easy for your body to absorb. If you're vegan, look for a plant-based blend that includes all essential amino acids.

- **Pay attention to the amount of protein per serving.** Look for products that deliver close to 30 grams of protein per serving.

- **Think about your lifestyle.** If you want to add protein to coffee, yogurt, or smoothies, an unflavored powder can be easier to work with and more versatile. If you're constantly on the go, you may do better with a premixed protein shake you can grab on your way out the door instead of a powder (or in addition to it!).

Getting the Hang of Monitoring Your Protein Intake

When it comes to protein, one of the biggest lightbulb moments happens at your first follow-up appointment as you and your provider look at your latest body composition report. This is when you'll begin to see the difference that protein makes, not just in how you feel but in your muscle retention. In other words—you can start to see what your daily protein intake has (or more likely, hasn't) done to your muscle.

It's a common scenario: A patient tells me they're hitting their protein target, but their body composition scan shows that they're losing muscle mass. Nine times out of ten, the discrepancy happens because they *think* they're getting enough protein, but they've either forgotten one of the guidelines described earlier or underestimated what 30 grams of protein looks like. When patients see the data in the body composition report, they begin to grasp the direct correlation between hitting their daily protein intake goal and muscle preservation.

Whether you're still waiting for your first follow-up appointment or you've already gone to it, it's important to track your day-to-day protein intake, especially at the beginning of your journey, when you haven't yet gotten the hang of estimating portion sizes and learned to check labels with a critical eye. Take time to sit down with a pen and paper and walk yourself through your day. Counting each serving of protein (and keeping in mind everything you're learning in this chapter as you do so) will help you learn the skills that will serve you well on your GLP-1 journey a lot more quickly.

A Day in the Life: An Example of a Protein-Packed Routine

On the pages that follow are some examples of what one day's food intake might look like. The snapshots that follow are not meant to be prescriptive meal plans or a mandate to eat six times a day; I just want to show you that 100+ grams of protein can fit into a normal schedule in several different ways. Your day can look however you want it to—the only principle to follow is prioritizing your protein intake; the rest of your plate is yours to customize. The key to success is intentionality: front-loading your protein, using efficient add-ins, and having a rhythm that works with your energy, appetite patterns, and lifestyle.

In the examples below, you'll see some meals that contain *more* than 30 grams of protein. That's fine—your body will use those extra nutrients in other ways—but remember that we'll only *count* 30 grams at a time toward your daily protein total. And please keep in mind: The protein guidelines that come along with a GLP-1 prescription are *not* a "diet" to help you lose weight but an essential part of preserving and building your muscle mass. With GLP-1 medication decreasing your appetite, you want to get the most out of your appetite for proper nutrition, and **protein must come first.**

Example 1

6:30 a.m.: Protein shake: **30 grams**

10:00 a.m.: 5 ounces grilled chicken with salad: **25 grams**

5:30 p.m.: 5 ounces grilled salmon with veggies: **30 grams**

8:30 p.m.: Protein pudding (made with 1 cup yogurt and 1 scoop chocolate whey protein isolate): **30 grams**

Total: **115 grams** of protein

Example 2

9:00 a.m.: Egg white omelet (5 egg whites and 1 ounce cheese): **25 grams**

12:00 p.m.: 1 cup cottage cheese and 4 ounces turkey meat: **25 grams**

3:00 p.m.: Protein shake: **25 grams**

6:00 p.m.: 4-ounce grilled steak with veggies: **25 grams**

Total: **100 grams** of protein

Example 3

8:00 a.m.: Chia pudding made with 6–8 ounces soy milk plus a scoop of whey protein powder: **35 grams**

12:00 p.m.: 1½ cups lentil soup with 2 tablespoons hemp hearts and 1 tablespoon nutritional yeast: **25 grams**

4:00 p.m.: Protein shake (pea protein isolate): **30 grams**

7:30 p.m.: 6 ounces baked tofu with peanut sauce over brown rice: **30 grams**

Total: 120 grams of protein

Example 4

7:30 a.m.: Overnight oats with protein powder: **30 grams**

11:30 a.m.: Taco salad bowl (with 4 ounces ground turkey): **30 grams**

3:00 p.m.: Protein shake: **30 grams**

7:00 p.m.: 4 scallops and sweet potato: **30 grams**

Total: 120 grams of protein

Example 5

7:00 a.m.: Protein shake: **30 grams**

12:30 p.m.: 5 ounces salmon with roasted vegetables: **25 grams**

4:00 p.m.: 1½ cups edamame: **20 grams**

7:00 p.m.: 5 ounces ground bison meat with ½ cup rice or pasta: **30 grams**

Total: 105 grams of protein

Example 6

7:00 a.m.: Protein smoothie with ½ cup Greek yogurt, 6–8 ounces milk, and one scoop protein powder: **30 grams**

10:30 a.m.: 1 cup cottage cheese: **14 grams**

2:00 p.m.: Lentil and farro bowl with 1 cup lentils, ½ cup farro, and 2 tablespoons pumpkin seeds: **25 grams**

7:00 p.m.: Tofu stir-fry (with 6 ounces tofu) and quinoa: **30 grams**

Total: 99 grams of protein

Example 7

7:00 a.m.: Protein coffee (blended with 1 scoop whey protein isolate): **30 grams**

12:00 p.m.: 6 ounces grilled steak with sweet potatoes: **45 grams**

5:00 p.m.: 6 ounces red snapper (or any fish) with ½ cup of grilled veggies: **30 grams**

8:30 p.m.: 1 cup cottage cheese with blueberries: **14 grams**

Total: 104 grams of protein

Patient-Tested Protein Tactics

Now that you have the guidelines to follow, let's talk about putting them into practice. For most people, this way of eating (prioritizing protein, spacing meals, paying attention to grams of protein) is a major lifestyle shift. I wish I could tell you that it's easy, but it's not. But isn't that the case with everything that is worth doing? What I *can* tell you is that with planning and discipline, you can get into a routine where it feels natural. Here are some of the most effective strategies I see patients using consistently. Choose a few that work for your routine and go from there.

- **Keep it convenient.** Find a ready-to-drink protein shake you like, and stock your fridge with it. I recommend having a premade option when you're on the go for convenience and consistency, and making homemade protein shakes when you're at home. Pro tip: Use an inexpensive handheld frother to quickly and easily blend protein powder without clumping.

- **Upgrade your coffee.** Add a scoop of protein powder to your morning coffee; it's a simple way to boost your intake without adding another meal. Whey protein isolate formulations tend to work best for this; plant-based protein powders can clump or have a gritty texture.
- **Protein + Greek yogurt = power snack.** Mix a scoop of protein powder into plain Greek yogurt and stir well. It becomes thick, creamy, and even more satisfying.
- **Sneak it in.** Stir unflavored protein powder into soups or sauces; it's an unnoticeable way to "up" the protein power of a meal.
- **Choose high-protein snacks.** Keep easy snacks on hand, such as hard-boiled eggs, cottage cheese, jerky, tuna packets, and roasted edamame.
- **Choose protein-forward carbs.** Opt for high-protein wraps, breads, or pastas (such as chickpea or lentil pasta) to sneak in more protein.
- **Prep ahead.** Make protein muffins, egg bites, or mini-meatballs ahead of time and freeze them; they are easy to grab and go.
- **Consume protein before bedtime.** Consider drinking a casein-based shake or Greek yogurt before bed to support overnight muscle repair. Casein is digested slowly, releasing amino acids for hours while you sleep.

If the information in this section feels overwhelming, that's okay. You don't have to remember all the amino acids to succeed (and there's no quiz at the end, I promise!). The point is for you to understand the importance of nutrition while you are on a GLP-1.

S Is for Strength Training

If you've completed your first assignment and increased your protein intake, you'll turn to strength training next. This is where many patients get excited. They've just started GLP-1 treatment, they're seeing some early changes, and they're eager to speed things up by hitting the gym. And I get it—there's nothing wrong with wanting to be proactive. But here's where I give them some counterintuitive advice: Yes, absolutely, move your body! Exercise is good. *But don't do it for the weight loss.*

I want you to pause here and let that sink in. Read it twice if you need to. **You need to exercise but not for weight loss.**

This might go against everything you've ever been told, but with GLP-1s, you need to reframe the way you've been conditioned to think about exercise. For—well—*forever*, people trying to lose weight have been told to exercise more. Run more. Burn more. Earn your food. Now you're using a medication that will do the heavy lifting on fat loss and body recomposition. This means that you don't need to exercise to make the scale drop faster.

Exercise now has a different purpose: to protect the progress that medication alone can't secure by keeping your body functional and strong. It's one of the most efficient, scalable, and effective ways to support your long-term health while using GLP-1s.

If thinking this way feels foreign to you, you're not alone. Maybe you've never lifted weights or done a push-up. Maybe just the words *strength training* make your brain flash to an image of heading to a CrossFit gym at 6:00 a.m. every day before work, and you already feel exhausted. But don't worry; you don't need to overhaul your lifestyle overnight. You just need an open mind and a willingness to take baby steps.

What Counts as Strength Training?

Strength training is a form of **resistance training**—any kind of movement where your muscles are working against a force. That force might be from a dumbbell, your bodyweight (as in push-ups and squats), a resistance band, or a machine, as long as it's making your muscles **contract against it**. Over time, resistance training tells your body, "This muscle tissue matters. Keep it!" It not only builds muscle but also extends endurance and improves bone density.

Strength training increases your **maximum force output**—in simpler terms, how much weight you can safely and consistently lift.

Strength workouts typically involve heavier weights and fewer repetitions per set. **The weight you're working with should be heavy enough** to make it very challenging to complete more than six to eight reps in a row. The general rule is: heavier weights, fewer reps; lighter weights, more reps. Because you're lifting heavier, you'll need longer rest periods between sets (around sixty to ninety seconds) to let your muscles recover before the next set.

A typical strength training workout might include several different exercises (such as squats, rows, or chest presses), each performed for three to five sets. You'll move through each set focusing on maintaining proper form, breathing, and gradually increasing the resistance over time. This progressive challenge is what builds muscle. The more you engage your muscles this way, the more metabolically active, resilient, and functional they will become—and the more muscle you will build.

One of the best things about strength training is how adaptable it is. You don't need expensive equipment or a gym membership to get started. You can get started with just your bodyweight or a few resistance bands. And because strength workouts often involve fewer reps and longer rest periods, they might take less time than high-rep classes or cardio routines to complete, making them particularly helpful for people with busy schedules or limited energy.

MY STORY WITH STRENGTH TRAINING

In my medical training, conversations about nutrition and physical activity were always front and center. Back then, they were the foundation for managing weight and preventing chronic conditions such as diabetes (and really, they were the *only* tools we had). Early on in my career, I realized something important: If I wanted to connect with my patients in a meaningful way, I would need to walk the walk.

That was when I started lifting weights and making protein intake a real priority in my own meals. Of course, I had always *logically* known how important muscle maintenance is. But knowing something and *doing* it are two very different things.

Once I began strength training, I understood it in a whole new way. It's not glamorous. It's not instant. It's real work. It means showing up on days when you're tired, sticking with it when you feel like giving up, and having the patience to progress slowly. I also learned that you can't just go through the motions; you have to learn the correct techniques. Early on in my training I tore a large muscle in my back. It was incredibly painful and set me back a full four weeks. But I got through it, kept going, and, most important, learned not to rush. Lifting weights has given me benefits that extend far beyond the gym. It's made me better at my job. I was no longer just sharing guidelines from a textbook; I was living them, feeling the benefits (and frustrations) firsthand.

If you're feeling nervous about adding strength training to your life, I can tell you with full honesty: I get it. I know it's not always convenient or exciting. But when you're on a GLP-1, protecting your muscle isn't just helpful—it's necessary.

How Strength Training Helps Muscle Grow

Any resistance-based movement is better than none, but strength training—using progressively heavier loads—is the most efficient way to preserve and build muscle. Of all the movement options available to you, strength training is the one most closely linked with improved metabolic health and physical function, injury prevention, and long-term weight maintenance. It provides the greatest return on investment for preserving and building muscle because it delivers more mechanical tension than lighter forms of resistance training, which makes it particularly effective for stimulating muscle growth. In other words, the more your muscles are safely pushed to handle heavier loads, the louder you're telling your body, "This muscle tissue matters to me. Keep it!"

During a strength training workout, you apply stress to your muscles and cause microscopic damage to them, often referred to as microtears. These tiny tears happen when your muscles are challenged with resistance they aren't fully used to. This damage is a good thing! It signals your body to repair, rebuild, and adapt. **When your body goes to work rebuilding**, it doesn't just repair those microtears; it reinforces the muscle at the site, making it slightly stronger and more resilient than before. That's how strength training leads to hypertrophy, or muscle growth, over time.

If you're still feeling intimidated, know that you don't have to start with barbells or big lifts. Resistance training can begin with bodyweight exercises and teach you how to "push" your muscles. You can build on that foundation by gradually increasing what your muscles can handle, finding out how much you can "push" with strength training. Both require time, patience, and discipline—but the rewards go far beyond the gym. Once you feel your strength building—you are lifting heavier, standing steadier, falling less, trusting your body more—you'll feel capable of doing anything, and you'll never want to go back. And remember: The more muscle you build, the more fat you burn and the more likely you are to maintain your weight loss long term, potentially on a much lower dose of a GLP-1.

Sleep and Recovery: Where the Magic Happens

Here's something most people don't realize: **Muscle doesn't grow in the gym; it grows when you rest.**

Yes, lifting weights is the stimulus, but the real transformation happens *afterward*, when your body has the time, fuel, and environment it needs to repair what you just challenged. That's where sleep comes in.

I'm sure you already know about the importance of sleep and all the reasons people usually prioritize it. Good sleep is great for supporting your GLP-1 journey: It helps regulate appetite, blood sugar, and stress levels and improves recovery from inflammation, but many people don't realize how crucial it is for muscle development, too.

When you're asleep (especially in the deeper stages of sleep), your body releases growth hormone, shuttles nutrients to your tissues, and gets to work repairing the microtears caused by your workout. This isn't just a "bonus" feature of sleep; it's a necessary part of the muscle-building process. Without adequate rest, your body can't rebuild what you broke down.

Rest is not just about sleep, though. You also need to **rest between workouts**. Strength training creates a temporary stress on the body; that's part of what makes it effective. But working the same muscle groups without adequate recovery time can lead to stalled progress, fatigue, and increased risk of injury.

So yes: Lift heavy. But then **get out of your own way** and let your body do what it knows how to.

Starting Safely

Over time, you'll naturally see progress with strength training—adding more resistance or trying new movements as your confidence and strength grow. But you don't need to rush that process. If you've never lifted weights before, I want you to hear this loud and clear: **Go slow, start small, and learn the basics.**

When GLP-1s start working, many patients start feeling better quickly and get a big rush of motivation to do everything possible to speed up their results. I know how exciting it can feel to finally be making progress, especially after years of frustration. But remember that when you are on GLP-1 treatment, you are a tortoise, not a hare. There's nothing you can (or should) do to speed up the process. This is all about staying strong (or getting stronger).

Injury is one of the most common reasons people abandon resistance training. And almost always, it happens because they are using poor form or lifting too much too soon. That's why getting started safely is so important. The following tips will help you build a strong, injury-free foundation so that your strength training will have results.

- **Take a few minutes to warm up and cool down.** Before you start lifting, do a few minutes of light movement such as walking or dynamic stretching to loosen your joints and get your blood flowing. After your workout, give yourself a few minutes to cool down and stretch. These small steps can help prevent injury and improve flexibility.
- **If possible, work with a personal trainer.** When you're starting out, I strongly recommend working with a personal trainer at the beginning—ideally in person. It doesn't need to be a lifelong commitment; even just a few sessions can make a huge difference in teaching you technique and helping you build a strong foundation. If a few starter sessions with a trainer are out of your budget, look for beginner strength classes in your area or small-group programs at local gyms or community centers. Some virtual programs can be helpful, too. It's always best to have a trainer who can watch you closely in real time and provide corrections when necessary, but if a virtual trainer is the best option for you now, it beats starting on your own.
- **Don't lift heavy weights on day one.** You're not lifting to impress anyone or become a "gym bro"; you're lifting to preserve your function, strength, and long-term health. Start with very light weights or even just your bodyweight (aka work without free weights, such as dumbbells) so that you can focus on good technique first. At this stage, you're just building the foundation. It may not feel like "real" strength training yet, but learning basic movements with control and intention is the first step. All strength training falls under the umbrella of resistance training; you're just starting at the most approachable end of the spectrum. You must gradually build strength in order

to begin resistance training with heavy weights. Weight lifting is a game of *patience*, just like GLP-1 therapy. Building strength takes time, and that's okay. It isn't a goal for you to conquer; it's a skill to practice continually.
- **Remember that protein is your fuel.** Your body can rebuild muscle only if it has the raw materials it needs. That's where good nutrition comes in. Remember, if your protein intake is low, your body can't fully repair the microtears in your muscle—and if you're also in a calorie deficit, it may even break down existing muscle to compensate.
- **Don't forget rest days.** I recommend strength training two to three nonconsecutive days per week for most beginners. It gives your body time to adapt between sessions.
- **If you miss a workout, don't panic.** Life happens, and sometimes you'll miss a workout. Strength is built over weeks and months, not days. Missing one session won't erase your progress, and it doesn't mean you're failing. Consistency over time, not perfection, is the key. If you can pick up where you left off and focus on the big picture, that's what really counts.

....

YOUR MUSCLES DON'T FORGET

If you ever fall off track for more than a few days or ever longer, don't assume that you're restarting from scratch. Once you've built strength, your muscles "remember" how to return to where they were faster than they did the first time. This is called muscle memory, and it's your body's way of adapting efficiently to familiar stresses. Whether you miss a week while traveling or take a longer break during a crazy period of your life, your progress will be more durable than you think. When you're ready, you can ease back in—and your body should meet you more than halfway.

....

NARA'S STORY

By the time I turned fifty, I felt like I had lost all control over my body. In the eighteen months leading up to that milestone birthday, I had gained forty pounds—despite everything I knew and practiced as a lifelong athlete.

At the same time, I was navigating late-stage perimenopause, recovering from a tough case of covid, running my own law practice, and raising three teenagers—and all with a family history of diabetes and obesity. The weight gain affected my energy, my confidence, and my ability to show up fully in my own life. I didn't feel like me anymore.

Despite seeking help from multiple medical professionals, I kept hearing the same message: *This is your new normal.* I was told to accept it as just a part of aging. The worst part was that no one believed me when I said I was already doing everything right.

Before giving in to that "new normal," I decided to seek out a provider—Dr. Rocio Salas-Whalen, who was experienced in prescribing GLP-1s for women struggling during perimenopause. That's when I started using Zepbound. Over the next several months, the weight began to come off steadily and consistently. For the first time in years, my body responded to my efforts. I had energy again. My blood pressure normalized. My labs improved. I began to see the return of the muscle I had worked so hard to build. Most important, I've significantly reduced my risk of developing the chronic diseases that run in my family.

Zepbound didn't replace discipline for me; it *unlocked* it. It allowed me to focus on body composition, not just the number on the scale. I prioritized protein, lifted heavier, stopped punishing myself, and started working *with* my physiology, not against it.

Eighteen months later, I'm over forty pounds down, stronger than I've been in years, and finally living in a body that feels like mine again—with the added confidence that I've taken real steps to protect my long-term health.

Reaching Your Destination

By now I hope you've realized that yes, this journey will ask something of you. You'll need to be consistent. You'll need to learn how to monitor your protein intake and prioritize your muscles as never before. But in return, you'll finally see real, sustainable results. Armed with knowledge and equipped with these nutrition strategies, you'll feel more energized, preserve your muscle, and protect your progress.

This doesn't mean you need to take extreme measures. You don't have to fight your way through hunger pangs or spend hours chasing gains in the gym. This time, your effort doesn't have to consume your life. Instead, you can focus on what actually works: fueling and challenging your body in the right ways and letting your medication work with your biology, not against it.

These recommendations about nutrition and exercise would benefit anyone, but when you are on a GLP-1, they are non-negotiable. They will help you achieve the bare minimum—preserving the muscle you have—and work toward the real win: building more strength, resilience, function, and, most important, confidence. These are the changes that will carry you forward in the long haul.

That's where your GPS comes into play. It's not just a metaphor but a guidepost you can return to whenever the road ahead feels unclear. Along with GLP-1s, protein intake and strength training are your anchors. Following your GPS can guarantee you an almost perfect journey—even when life gets chaotic and even when progress slows.

There will be detours and days when things feel off course. That's normal; in fact, that's life. But for the first time, you won't just be along for the ride; you'll be in the driver's seat. Now that your biology is working with you, every step you take will move you forward.

The road ahead won't always be smooth, but what matters most is that you *keep going.*

CHAPTER 7

Titration and Troubleshooting: Adjusting Your Dose and Navigating Side Effects

Before we dive into this chapter, I want to take a moment to tell you how proud I am of you. There has been a lot to take in—new information, new habits, new ways of thinking about health and weight—and you're still here, showing up for yourself. That matters more than you know.

Now it's time to fine-tune your treatment. Titration, the gradual adjustment of your GLP-1 dose, is not a setback or something to push through; it's a built-in part of your treatment and is something that the majority of patients using these medications will need to do at some point in their journey. These medications are designed to evolve with your body, and adjusting your dose over time helps ensure that they will keep working as effectively as possible.

In this chapter, you'll learn how the titration process works: when and why your dose might need to increase and in some cases when it might need to decrease. You'll also get practical guidance for troubleshooting common issues that can come up during treatment. Don't worry, most of your journey will be smooth sailing, especially if you follow my recommendations closely.

Fine-Tuning Your Treatment with Titration

When it comes to GLP-1 treatment, titration is one of the most important parts of your journey. Unlike many medications that stay fixed at one dose, GLP-1s typically require careful, ongoing adjustment to stay effective. Think of each dose as having an "expiration date" in effectiveness. For most people, the benefits of a given dose begin to level off after about three months. When that happens, it may be time to increase your dose in order to continue seeing results. This pattern likely reflects a combination of factors. Based on years of clinical experience, I've observed that each dose level tends to deliver a certain amount of weight to lose; it's common to require higher doses to continue progressing. In some cases, patients may also develop a degree of tolerance, meaning that the appetite-suppressing effects that were strong at first start to wear off, even if the same dose once worked well. When this happens, it means it may be time for an upward adjustment.

Generally speaking, if your goal is to achieve body recomposition by losing about twenty pounds, you'll likely only need the first or second dose to reach it. But if you need to lose thirty pounds or more to improve your metabolic health, you'll probably need to move through most or all of the available dose levels. And that's where the experience of your provider becomes especially important.

That said, there is no one-size-fits-all process for titration.

Some people stay on the starting dose for longer than three months. Some never need to go beyond it. Like everything else with GLP-1 therapy, what this part of the journey looks like will depend on the individual. There are no rigid guidelines or perfect formulas for when and how to increase your dose. What I'm sharing with you here is based on what I've seen work for thousands of patients in my clinic.

Slow and Steady

Here are a few reasons why gradual titration is important.

- **You avoid "maxing out" on your medication.** If your weight loss goal is fifty pounds or more, it's important to make the most of each dose level before moving up. In other words, give each dose a full opportunity to work while it still feels effective. Rushing through the titration schedule too quickly can leave you at the highest available dose before you've reached your target without anywhere left to go. (More on this in the sidebar on pages 160 to 161.)
- **You help your body tolerate larger doses.** Increasing your doses gradually prepares your body for the stronger appetite suppression of the higher doses later on. In fact, you don't want to increase your dose unless you're tolerating your current dose well, with minimal or manageable side effects. Otherwise, the side effects of the next dose up will be much worse.
- **You avoid rapid muscle loss.** If your appetite drops dramatically overnight, you risk severe caloric restriction—and that's when muscle loss happens. You might see the number on the scale plummet. But losing muscle is not success. Muscle protects your metabolism, insulin sensitivity, and long-term weight stability. Remember: Preserve your muscle mass at all costs.

- **You have time to learn to hit your protein targets.** Consuming 90 to 100 grams of protein per day is challenging even without appetite suppression. Moving too fast into higher doses makes it even harder to meet your protein needs. We want you to practice and master your protein intake early, when your appetite is still on the stronger side.
- **You give every dose a fair shot.** GLP-1 medications are designed to be long-acting. Remember that our own GLP-1 lasts only two to four minutes before it is broken down. GLP-1 analogs, on the other hand, last anywhere from twenty-four hours to seven days.
- **You avoid changing your dosage before your body is ready.** This way, you will have a lower likelihood of wasting valuable medication.

Extending the Time Between Dose Increases

For patients with significant weight loss goals (sixty, eighty, one hundred pounds or more), spending more time at each dose is important. Otherwise, you might be taking the highest dose available but be only partway through your weight loss journey and with nowhere else to go. Semaglutide has a total of five dose levels, tirzepatide has six, and liraglutide typically follows a daily escalation up to five doses: 0.6, 1.2, 1.8, 2.4, and 3.0 milligrams. We need to make each dose last as long as it's still working. This doesn't mean staying at a dose if your appetite suppression wears off or your fat loss stalls; those are clear signs that it's time to move up. But if your dose is still doing its job, don't rush to the next one. If you burn through all your doses too quickly, you might run out of therapeutic options before reaching your target.

At the time of writing, semaglutide at a whopping dose of 7.2 milligrams is being researched in a phase IIIb study (in clinical trials). So far, the results show that this higher dose leads to about 10 percent more weight loss than the current 2.4-milligram dose.

When and Why to Titrate Up

In general, your current dose should have an effect for two to three months before its effects start to plateau. As your body adjusts to GLP-1 therapy, there may come a time when your current dose isn't quite getting the job done. There are two key signs it might be time to increase.

1. **Appetite suppression doesn't last a full seven days at your current dose.** This means that real hunger (not just appetite or eating out of habit) returns well before your next injection. The appetite suppression should feel consistent from one injection to the next. And no, you should not take your next injection early; what you need is a higher dose.

2. **Your weight plateaus for several weeks, and your body composition analysis shows that you're no longer losing fat.** A higher dose may be needed to reengage your metabolic response.

If either of these scenarios is happening, get in touch with your doctor to discuss if it may be time to increase your dosage.

When and Why to Titrate Down

Titration isn't always about moving upward; in certain circumstances, lowering your dose may be more important than increasing it.

- **You're struggling with side effects.** If you're already uncomfortable at your current dose, pushing higher will only make things worse. Lowering the dose may help stabilize you, prevent dropout, and keep you moving forward.

CAN NAUSEA HELP WITH WEIGHT LOSS?

Patients on older versions of GLP-1, such as exenatide, liraglutide, and even semaglutide, tend to experience more nausea than those on tirzepatide. Occasionally, this leads them to switch to tirzepatide—only to come back a few weeks later saying that it didn't "work" the same because they notice the return of food noise or old eating habits. In my experience, some subtle discomfort from semaglutide—which some patients report as nausea—can play a helpful role in appetite suppression. For certain patients, that subtle discomfort may be part of what helps them be more mindful of how much they are eating. Please note that I'm talking only about a sensation that feels similar to an uncomfortable fullness. If the nausea is more severe or there is vomiting, this is not "subtle," and you need to consult your doctor.

- **You need to protect your muscle.** If you're losing weight too rapidly, you're almost certainly losing muscle, too. As discussed earlier, preserving muscle trumps all. Muscle is your metabolism's best friend. Losing it slows your fat loss, lowers your energy, and impedes your long-term success. You may need to lower your dose for the greater good of preserving your muscle.
- **You need help to hit your protein goal.** If the appetite-suppressing effects of your medication make it hard for you to hit 90 to 100 grams of protein daily, that's a major problem. In this case, lowering the dose of your medication will be the best option for preserving muscle mass. Sometimes lowering the dose slightly rather than

forcing it allows you to eat enough to support your muscle—and your overall results.

Troubleshooting: What to Do When Progress Stalls

Now that you understand the principle of titration, let's talk about one of the most common reasons you may need to adjust your dose: the fat loss plateau. This can be a frustrating and even scary moment for many patients. You've been doing everything right, and then suddenly the scale stops moving. Before you panic, let me tell you this: It does not mean that the medication isn't working or that you're doing something wrong.

Is It Actually a Weight Plateau?

As I mentioned before, every dose has an "expiration date," and for most people, that's around three months. After that point, the same dose may not be as effective, and your weight loss may slow down or stall. But sometimes what you're seeing is due not to stalled fat loss but to new muscle being built. Yes, you read that right; since muscle is denser than fat, it takes up less space but weighs more. So if you're gaining muscle while losing fat, your weight might stay the same for a while. That's why the number on the scale can be misleading: You may be making major progress with body recomposition, even if it doesn't show up as a drop in pounds. That's why it's important to look beyond the scale and dig into what's actually happening in your body. Here's how to tell whether you're truly in a fat loss plateau or it's just that the number on the scale is not telling you the full story.

Step One: Check Your Body Composition

If your weight has plateaued, the very first thing to do is conduct another body composition analysis.

- **If your fat loss has slowed and you're maintaining muscle,** it's time to increase your dose.
- **If your muscle mass is dropping but your fat percentage isn't,** it's time to revisit your protein intake (see step two). You might need to consider decreasing your dose, too.

Step Two: Assess Your Protein Intake

Many patients unknowingly overestimate how much protein they're getting. If your intake is insufficient or your medication dose is too strong, suppressing your appetite too much, you'll start losing muscle. No matter what, preserving muscle is nonnegotiable. If you're losing muscle, you first need to confirm whether you're truly hitting your protein targets. Ask yourself these questions.

- Am I spreading my daily protein intake across four servings?
- Am I choosing high-quality, complete proteins?
- Am I adjusting my schedule based on satiety cues?

If you're doing everything right with protein and still struggling, keep reading.

Step Three: Look Deeper

If your protein intake is solid, your dose is stable, and you're still struggling to lose fat, it may be time to investigate further. By now you know that GLP-1s work with your biology, but your biology is unique to you. And in some cases, your body may need more support than GLP-1s alone can offer.

- **Metabolic assessment:** Not every person's body responds to a medication in the same way. Some patients have a naturally slow metabolism due to aging, hormonal imbalances, low muscle mass, or simply individual variation. And when your baseline metabolism is very slow, weight loss can stall or not progress as expected, even with the help of a GLP-1 agonist. Others may have more weight to lose, especially those with a goal of losing a hundred pounds or more. In these cases, your doctor may consider combination therapy with another drug beyond your GLP-1, such as Qsymia. Qsymia is a non-GLP-1 prescription medication that combines low doses of phentermine and topiramate, and it's FDA approved for chronic weight management. The goal isn't just to "add more" medication, but to extend the effectiveness of each dose of your GLP-1. A second medication can help preserve your response to the GLP-1 agonist for longer, preventing the need to escalate your dose too quickly.

    Before tirzepatide came onto the market, I almost always started patients with significant weight loss goals on Qsymia simultaneously with semaglutide. Now that newer GLP-1 medications are more sophisticated and efficient, combination therapy may become less common. But for now, in certain cases, it's still the most effective path forward.

- **Genetic testing:** Rare monogenic mutations, such as POMC or MC4R mutations, can slow weight loss despite optimal treatment. Obesity caused by these mutations often presents in early childhood, but some people with milder variants of these mutations may not be aware of them until they are well into adulthood. These genetic variations interfere with normal hunger, satiety, and weight regulation. Two of the most studied examples are mutations in the POMC (pro-opiomelanocortin) and MC4R (melanocortin 4 receptor) genes.

1. **POMC mutations** can disrupt how the brain signals fullness, making it much harder to regulate food intake.
2. **MC4R mutations,** one of the most common genetic contributors to severe obesity, affect energy balance and appetite control.

Needing combination therapy or additional tools isn't a reflection of your effort, your willpower, or your worth. It's simply the reality that weight regulation is complex and sometimes other factors need to be addressed. But we now have tools and treatments that can address these complex factors—tools that didn't exist even a few years ago.

Appetite Changes

There's one more variable that deserves your attention: your appetite. When you are on a GLP-1, your appetite will change in ways you really have to experience to understand. This is part of how the medication works, of course, but it can create new challenges. Some people may find it difficult to muster up enough appetite to eat enough to support their body's needs. For others, hunger seems to return sooner than expected. Neither scenario means that the medication is failing, but both are worth addressing.

If You're Not Hungry Enough to Eat

Some patients find that their appetite becomes *too* suppressed—so much that they struggle to meet their protein target or forget to eat altogether, which can lead to headaches, nausea, or feeling weak. This happens most commonly in the early stages of treatment or right after you've gone up a dose. If this is a challenge for you, here's how you can handle it.

- **Stick to small high-protein meals** (see the Protein Cheat Sheet on page 228 for ideas and inspiration).
- **Make sure to leave enough time between meals and shakes,** so they don't replace each other.
- **Try eating on a schedule** rather than waiting to feel hungry.
- **Front-load your protein earlier in the day,** when your appetite may be stronger.

If Your Hunger Returns Early

Sometimes patients notice their appetite creeping back before their next injection is due. If this happens to you, don't ignore it; this is exactly the kind of feedback your provider needs to hear to guide your next steps. In the meantime, keep your protein intake high to help maintain satiety. If real hunger returns early, consider it useful information. Listen to your body, choose nourishing, protein-rich foods, and jot down what you're noticing. Together with your provider, you can determine whether a dose adjustment is the right move. Staying attuned to your appetite shifts is one of the most valuable tools you have. These changes are how your body communicates, and sharing them helps your care team keep you on track in a sustainable, effective way.

Managing Side Effects

Every medication has side effects. Even common over-the-counter medications can cause serious harm if misused or taken in the wrong circumstances. Whenever a doctor prescribes a medication, the decision always comes down to a careful evaluation of this question: Do the benefits of the medication outweigh the risks from its side effects?

When it comes to GLP-1s, the answer is overwhelmingly "yes." The health risks associated with untreated obesity—diabetes, heart disease, stroke, cancer—are far more common and far more dangerous than the side effects of GLP-1 therapy.

That said, it's important to be well informed. You should always know the possible risks and side effects of any medication you're considering, read the information that comes with the medication, and never hesitate to discuss your concerns with your doctor. You should feel confident in your care, and your doctor's goal should always be to maximize benefits while minimizing risks. Let's take a closer look at GLP-1s' side effects together.

Common Side Effects

Side effects are common with *any* drug; even over-the-counter medications can have serious side effects. The reason a medication gets FDA approval is not that it has no side effects but that the positive benefits of the drug are greater than the possibility of serious side effects occurring. This is why I strongly recommend FDA-approved GLP-1 medications. Most of the side effects of GLP-1s tend to be mild and non–life threatening; this is one of the reasons we can prescribe them.

Most of the side effects of any medication are dose dependent. Typically, the higher the dose, the more likely side effects are to occur; the lower the dose, the fewer side effects you'll experience.

GLP-1s' side effects vary widely among patients. Some people are very sensitive to nausea or constipation, while others notice barely any change. They're most likely to appear when you're first starting out or increasing your dose, and in many cases, they ease on their own as your body adjusts—often within a few days to a couple of weeks.

No matter what dose you're on, you should never feel as though you must put up with side effects while taking this medication. GLP-1s are meant to work with your body, not against it, and most side effects have solutions. Remember: *You don't have to suffer to lose weight.* If a side effect is severe or disruptive or lasts more than two weeks, it's a good idea to check in with your doctor. It's important to communicate openly with your doctor if you're struggling or questioning if something you're experiencing is indeed an associated side effect and can be managed. Here are some side effects that you can expect.

> **Nausea** is probably the most frequently reported side effect. It can be caused by the medication itself or, in some cases, by the unfamiliar sensation of early fullness. This is especially true for patients who are accustomed to needing larger meals to feel satisfied; your mind may not immediately "catch up" to your body's signals, and you may not feel as though you've already eaten beyond that natural stopping point. Always try to follow your instincts and be on the lookout for satiety cues from your body. Mealtime is over when your body signals fullness, not when your plate is empty.
>
> **What to do:** If you're having intense nausea on the first or second day after your injections and it feels like a hurdle you can't get over, ask your doctor if nausea medication may be a good idea for you. Because tirzepatide causes less nausea than semaglutide, in some cases, it may be worth speaking to your provider about switching meds.

MORNING NAUSEA AND HUNGER CONFUSION

If you feel nauseous first thing in the morning, consider when you last ate. Sometimes nausea is your body's way of signaling low blood sugar or an empty stomach—even if you don't consciously feel hunger. Try eating a small protein-rich meal to settle your stomach.

Diarrhea can occur with any class of GLP-1 medication, especially if you eat greasy, fried, or overly fatty foods while on treatment. Meals that are heavy in fat tend to pass through your digestive tract very quickly, leading to discomfort.

What to do: Call your doctor as soon as possible after diarrhea happens. Skip your next dose until you speak with your doctor or your symptoms resolve. If a patient is experiencing diarrhea, I don't recommend increasing the next dose until it has subsided and they can even consider decreasing to the lowest dose where any side effects were more tolerable. (The same advice applies if you're experiencing nausea.)

Constipation is common when on semaglutide, less so with tirzepatide. Because you'll be eating smaller meals, your overall intake of food and fiber naturally decreases. This slows digestion—and dehydration also contributes.

What to do: Increase your water intake, and consider adding a fiber supplement at bedtime if needed. If constipation is severe or persistent, discuss it with your doctor; you may need to adjust your medication or treatment plan.

Gas is a very common complaint from patients. Upper intestinal gas, which can cause lots of burping, is often linked to carbonated beverages such as soda or sparkling water. Gas bubbles can slow down digestion and increase discomfort. Lower intestinal gas, which can lead to bloating and flatulence, can also occur and be surprisingly painful. Bubbly beverages can also contribute to this, but the more common culprits are fiber-rich foods such as beans, lentils, and cruciferous vegetables. If a food is known for causing gas under normal circumstances, it's likely to cause even more when you are on a GLP-1. Your digestive system is more sensitive now, and what was mildly gas-inducing before may now feel amplified.

What to do: Cut back on carbonated drinks such as soda and sparkling water or ease up on fiber-rich foods such as beans, lentils, and cruciferous vegetables until your symptoms improve.

Dehydration can occur as a direct side effect of the medication, as some GLP-1s may slightly suppress thirst signals. Eating less frequently may also cause you to drink less without realizing it. It's very important to be proactive about hydration and drink even if you don't feel thirsty.

What to do: I strongly recommend that my patients add electrolytes to their water. They help the water "work" better for your body, so it can retain the fluids you drink and improve your overall hydration. Without adequate electrolytes, much of the water you drink is quickly lost through urine instead of being absorbed and used where it's needed. Electrolyte powders or tablets are usually a better choice than sports drinks, which tend to be more sugary. If your thirst cues are suppressed, try building hydration into your routine and keep a water bottle with you throughout the day. You can even set reminders on your phone, if needed.

Acid reflux is also a common side effect, especially in patients who had reflux or heartburn before starting GLP-1 treatment. Acid reflux while on a GLP-1 tends to occur more frequently during the night or while you're lying down. GLP-1s slow down gastric emptying, meaning that food stays in your stomach longer; that's part of how they keep you feeling full quicker and longer, but it also increases the risk of reflux if you lie down too soon after eating.

What to do: I usually recommend that my patients make their dinner the smallest meal and to leave at least two to three hours between eating and going to bed. Giving your body time to digest before lying flat can make a big difference in reducing nighttime discomfort.

Vomiting is never a normal or expected side effect of GLP-1s. That said, it can occasionally happen when someone significantly overeats past their new satiety threshold. This is especially common in situations where inhibition is lowered, such as after a night of drinking. Alcohol can make it easier to miss your body's fullness cues and can lead to choices (such as late-night pizza) that you might not have made otherwise. If vomiting happens spontaneously *without* overeating, it could signal a serious adverse event and should be taken seriously.

What to do: First, you need to stop your GLP-1. Never inject your next dose if you are vomiting. Otherwise, the vomiting will get worse and can be dangerous. Second, call your doctor and describe your symptoms. Because vomiting can lead to dehydration, drink fluids. Your doctor may prescribe a dose of anti-nausea medication, taken orally if you can tolerate it. If you can't keep the medication down, you may need to take it in the form of a suppository or an injection. To receive an injection, you most likely will need to go to urgent care.

Secondary Side Effects: Warning Signs

Some of the most commonly discussed "side effects" of GLP-1s are not actually caused by the medication itself; they're secondary side effects, often resulting from rapid weight loss, inadequate protein intake, or undereating. I think of them not as true side effects but as clues that your body needs more support during your GLP-1 journey. Catching them means that you can tweak your approach and keep moving forward, stronger than ever.

Headaches

- **Likely cause:** Dehydration, changes in eating patterns, or shifts in blood sugar.

- **What to do:** First, make sure you're drinking enough water; dehydration is a common cause of headaches when you are on a GLP-1. If you've recently changed your caffeine intake or eating schedule, those shifts could also contribute. If your headaches persist or worsen, talk to your doctor.

Muscle Loss

- **Likely cause:** Losing weight too quickly without adequate protein intake.

- **What to do:** This was covered extensively in chapter 6, but to recap, reassess your daily protein intake and spacing. Focus on strength training to preserve your lean muscle mass.

Hair Thinning or Shedding

- **Likely cause:** Nutrient depletion (for example, from low protein intake).

- **What to do:** Ensure that you're meeting your protein goal, staying nourished, and losing weight at a steady, sustainable pace.

Fatigue or Low Energy

- **Likely cause:** Insufficient calorie intake, low protein, dehydration, or nutrient gaps.

- **What to do:** Review your nutrition and hydration habits and try to pay closer attention to thirst or hunger cues. (See "Appetite Changes" on page 166 for more tips.)

Loose or Sagging Skin

- **Likely cause:** Rapid, unbalanced fat loss without muscle preservation.

- **What to do:** Focusing on a slower, steadier fat loss pace while building and preserving muscle underneath can help minimize loose skin.

Uncommon Side Effects

Most patients on GLP-1 therapy will never experience these side effects; they're rare. But because they are not nonexistent, it's important to be aware of them. Early recognition and timely action can make all the difference if anything does arise. Let's walk through the less common risks you should be aware of.

Pancreatitis

Pancreatitis is a rare but serious inflammation of the pancreas. This complication is more often seen in people with diabetes. For GLP-1s to stimulate the pancreas, there typically needs to be an abnormal elevated glucose level. In patients without diabetes, the pancreas is generally not stimulated by GLP-1s. That said, cases of pancreatitis have been reported in these patients, and they are serious enough to warrant your attention.

How will you know if it's happening? As I mentioned in chapter 3, pancreatitis is not the kind of thing that you sleep off at home or that goes away on its own. Symptoms typically include severe pain on your left flank just below your left ribs, often radiating to your back, along with severe nausea, vomiting, and feeling extremely unwell. It will be obvious that something's wrong. If this happens, go to the emergency room immediately.

Certain factors can increase your risk, including a history of gallstones, heavy alcohol use, or very high triglyceride levels. Eating a high-sugar diet while on a GLP-1 medication can also contribute to the overstimulation of the pancreas—another reason this medication should be used in partnership with thoughtful nutrition choices.

Gallbladder Issues (Cholelithiasis and Cholecystitis)

Gallstones (cholelithiasis) and gallbladder inflammation (cholecystitis) are rare but documented complications of GLP-1 use, especially in individuals with other known risk factors. These risk factors include having overweight or obesity, losing weight quickly, being female (especially during the childbearing years, although the risk continues to rise with age), or having a family history of gallbladder issues.

Any rapid weight loss, regardless of how it's achieved, increases the risk of gallstone formation, which is why we don't want to rush weight loss. But GLP-1 medications also slow down the contraction of the stomach and gallbladder, which can further increase the likelihood of developing a gallstone and even lead to gallbladder inflammation, especially if you already have a predisposition to these issues.

Signs of a potential gallbladder complication include pain in the upper right abdomen (especially after meals) that may radiate to the shoulder. If you experience this kind of pain regularly, your doctor may recommend an ultrasound to evaluate for gallstones or gallbladder inflammation.

Medullary Thyroid Carcinoma (MTC)

GLP-1 medications carry a boxed warning about medullary thyroid carcinoma, a very rare and aggressive form of thyroid cancer. This warning is based on findings from rodent studies, in which the medication was shown to accelerate tumor growth with this type of cancer (see chapter 2 for a discussion of this), but this has not been confirmed in humans. While the risk in humans appears to be extremely low, out of an abundance of caution, GLP-1s are not recommended for people with a personal or family history of MTC or multiple endocrine neoplasia syndrome type 2 (MEN2), which includes MTC.

If you have a history of any of these conditions or you're unsure if you do, talk to your doctor before starting GLP-1 therapy. Screening is straightforward, and contraindications are rare—but they should not be overlooked.

AMANDA'S STORY

I have always been someone who struggled with my weight in a family with people who didn't. It never really made sense to me. Why was I so dramatically different from everyone else? I ate the same things, worked out, and played sports, but I was always significantly heavier.

Aging hasn't made it any easier. I've lost and regained the same forty, fifty, sixty pounds since my early twenties. I've done all the programs and tried talking to doctors, but the advice is always the same. In 2017, I did extensive genetic testing that showed I had severe PCOS and insulin resistance.

While I was initially nervous to start Zepbound at age

forty-one—mostly because of misinformation about the side effects—its impact on my life has been nothing short of revelatory. The medication lets me feel normal for the first time in my life. I don't feel like I'm trying to white-knuckle through a highly restrictive diet plan every day, and it's incredibly freeing. I lost a hundred pounds in the first twelve months on Zepbound. My only regret is that I didn't start sooner.

Precision, Patience, and Progress

You've come so far already. By working through this chapter, you've armed yourself with the knowledge of how your body may respond to GLP-1 therapy. You've learned how to recognize when your dose is working, how to tell when it may need to change, and how to troubleshoot when something doesn't feel right.

In this part of your GLP-1 journey, your success will come down to three things: precision, patience, and progress. Each one plays a different role, and together they form the mindset that will carry you forward throughout the rest of your treatment.

Precision means learning to listen to your body (even the subtle shifts) and making smart, strategic adjustments based on that feedback. This skill will help you know when a side effect needs attention, when you may want to consult with your provider, and when things are working just fine.

Patience will keep you grounded when progress feels slow or nonlinear. Resist the urge to rush to a higher dose just to see the scale move faster. Your body needs time and support to adapt safely, and when you give it that time, it rewards you with more sustainable results; don't ever underestimate the power of stability.

Progress might look different than you expected. Maybe you're measuring it by your clothing size or the increasing amount of energy you have. Maybe it's simply learning to trust your hunger signals again. Progress doesn't have to be loud or dramatic to be real as long as you're still showing up and moving forward, even when it feels slow, even when it isn't perfectly linear.

This is *real* transformation—transformation that takes time. If you've made it through this chapter, you've proven that you can do hard things, and you're stronger for it. In the next chapter, you'll use this confidence and knowledge to navigate what happens next: maintaining your progress over time, whether you stay on your medication or decide to taper off.

PART III
Life After GLP-1s

CHAPTER 8

Maintaining Your Weight: Strategies for Sustained Success

What a journey—you made it! As I write this, I can't help but feel emotional thinking of all my patients who've stood where you are standing now. After months of treatment and hard work—and a lifetime of thinking that their health goals were impossible—they reached them. And now so have you. It's not an accident; it's not a dream. You've done more than lose the amount of weight recommended by your provider; you've changed your body composition and reduced your body fat percentage while preserving (or even building) muscle mass. You have positively impacted your energy, your metabolism, and your long-term health. It's a new reality; and you, my dear reader, achieved all this! This treatment plan isn't easy; it takes focus, effort, and consistency. I am so proud of the work you've done.

While this is an important milestone, you might already be wondering how you will maintain your current weight. You might even feel a little anxious about it. If so, please know that those feelings *are normal*. I see it in my patients: the fear of regaining weight, of letting go of the structure that got them to this point. On top of that, there's no shortage of fear-based messaging out there about taking GLP-1s long term: "Once you're on GLP-1s, you can never stop!" "You'll need to take them *forever*! For *eternity*!"

They're everywhere—sensationalized headlines, viral posts, scare tactics. And none of them is helpful. So let's clear the air and talk about what it will take to stay where you are. Welcome to maintenance.

Entering Weight Maintenance: What Happens Now?

Maintenance marks a major shift in how we approach your care. During the fat loss phase, your body operated in a caloric deficit; you were burning more energy than you consumed. That deficit made your body tap into its fat stores for fuel, gradually reducing your overall body fat. Now you've reached the fat loss targets defined by your unique body composition. Ideally, you maintained or even built muscle during that process. The goal is no longer to promote fat loss. Instead, you'll:

- Maintain your current weight
- Prevent body fat regain
- Rebuild muscle if there was muscle loss

To accomplish these new goals, you'll need to put new systems into place to protect your progress: physiologically, behaviorally, and emotionally. That includes examining how you use medication, train your body, fuel it, and respond to life's ongoing challenges.

Maintenance shouldn't feel as though it's consuming your life, but it's not something that happens passively, either. It requires staying engaged with your treatment in a new, more balanced way. You'll need to reinforce the habits that got you here and learn how to live with confidence in your new body.

Think of it this way: During the active fat loss phase, your GLP-1 medication played the leading role; it was doing much of the heavy lifting, helping regulate your appetite, reduce your cravings, and support your metabolic change. But now, in maintenance, the script shifts. The medication steps into a supporting role, still present and valuable but no longer at center stage. Now it's time for *you* to take the lead—and along with it more of the accountability for maintaining your healthy habits, strength, awareness, and consistency. Now you're stepping into your power and making the results from the medication yours to keep for a lifetime.

What Are Your Options for Maintenance?

For weight loss maintenance, there are two options: to continue with GLP-1 long term or to stop it. If you've followed my work, you already know where I stand. I strongly recommend that most patients continue the medication because obesity is a *chronic, multifactorial disease*. While GLP-1s do not *cure* it, they can *control* it.

In fact, supporting long-term maintenance might be the most powerful and revolutionary contribution that GLP-1 medications have to offer. I'll be honest: This is my favorite aspect of these medications. Think about how many diets you've tried over the years, how many extreme plans or restrictions you've strictly followed because they promised transformation—only to fall short when it came to maintenance. You may have even lost weight on some of those methods before, but it was probably not the right kind of weight loss. You might have just decreased the number on the scale, not necessarily lost *fat*. And once the diet plan ended, so did your progress.

GLP-1s disrupt this cycle. For the first time in medical history, we have medications that don't just support fat loss, they help people maintain it. At a lower (maintenance) dose, GLP-1s continue to support appetite regulation, reduce cravings, and slow gastric emptying—all of which make it easier to maintain a stable, reduced calorie intake without constantly fighting hunger. It doesn't replace your effort or habits, but it makes it easier to sustain them without having to rely on sheer willpower day after day.

In my practice, about 95 percent of patients choose to stay on treatment, even those who began their journey planning to stop it after reaching their goal. Why? Because once they understand the biology of obesity—and experience life without the constant "food noise" that tormented them for years—they realize that GLP-1s are a tool worth keeping. The small number of patients who choose to stop taking the medication often do so just to see how their body responds or for lifestyle or medical reasons.

Whatever your situation and no matter what choice you make, the next two sections will explore both options: what continuing medication looks like and what it takes to stop taking it safely and successfully. Let's start with what it looks like to stay on medication for the long term.

Obesity Is Chronic: The Case for Continuing Medication

As discussed in chapter 1, obesity is a chronic, multifactorial condition. Remember that "chronic" simply means that the condition isn't curable—but it *is* manageable. Obesity and its related risks can be controlled with the right tools and care. Think about high blood pressure, type 2 diabetes, or depression. We don't "cure" these conditions; we keep them in check, regulated, and controlled. The same is true here.

Even if you don't meet the criteria for obesity anymore or even if you never technically did, you may still have a physiological or environmental predisposition to weight gain. That predisposition doesn't necessarily disappear once you've reached a certain weight. The factors that play a role might have less influence, but for many patients, they will always be there. Many of you reading this have probably taken a ride or two on the dieting roller coaster. You hit your goal weight, only to feel it slipping away months later. That cycle of hope, success, excitement, regain, frustration, and disappointment is *painful*. So why, when we finally have something that interrupts that cycle, are we so quick to let people label long-term use of a medication a failure or a negative outcome?

Taking a GLP-1 medication is not failure; it's medical care.

I know that some of you are still wrestling with the idea of continuing medication. It's common and understandable. I invite you to pause and ask yourself this: Would you feel the same hesitation if this were a medication for your thyroid?

Imagine someone saying that they plan to stop their thyroid medication because their symptoms have improved and their labs look normal. Most people would immediately point out that their thyroid levels are normal *because of* the medication—and stopping it abruptly could cause symptoms to return. The logical next step would be to check with a doctor, not stop cold turkey.

Now imagine someone with depression saying that they feel better, so they're tossing their antidepressants. Again, we instinctively understand that *feeling better is a sign that the medication is working*—not a reason to abandon it without a plan.

The same principle applies to GLP-1s for weight loss and metabolic health. If you're feeling better, functioning better, and seeing real results, that's not a cue to quit; it's proof that the treatment is effective. In other words, **you shouldn't stop taking a medication for a chronic condition because it's working.**

Here's what I want you to keep remembering, especially now that you're entering maintenance: These medications are a form of ongoing treatment—part of a comprehensive plan to help you maintain what you've worked so hard to achieve. You and I know this. The problem is that we still struggle—as a society and as individuals—to accept obesity as a chronic medical condition. Wanting to lose weight is often seen as a superficial and cosmetic pursuit. For instance, we get "in shape" for a wedding or drop a dress size before a reunion. If that's the lens you're using, of course, staying on medication sounds extreme or unnecessary. You might hear people say, "Well, you lost the weight. Why keep taking it?" They may tell you that now that the weight loss is done, your treatment should be, too—as if the only goal was to fit into a smaller dress. That mindset misses the point entirely. This journey was never just about a number on the scale or a clothing size; it was about reclaiming your health, your energy, your confidence—your *life*.

If that's how you used to think before picking up this book, that's okay. It means you've grown and you now have a deeper understanding of your body, your biology, and what sustainable health truly looks like. With that understanding, you now have the power to share this knowledge and change the conversation for someone else who is still stuck in the old narrative.

GRACE'S STORY

During the pandemic, I held an incredibly demanding job as one of the people responsible for supervising the quality of over 100,000 meals a day for frontline workers and communities in need. The stress of that role took a serious toll on my health. I experienced a hormonal imbalance that led me to gain about twenty pounds. While that might not sound like much, for me, it was significant—and I didn't feel like myself.

Beyond the weight, I was constantly tired, low on energy, and struggling with mood swings. It was hard to keep up with the fast-paced lifestyle I'd always had as a chef—constantly traveling, always surrounded by food, and rarely on a routine.

When I finally went to see Dr. Rocio Salas-Whalen, she suggested I consider a GLP-1 medication. It turned out to be one of the best decisions I've ever made. Not only did I lose the weight, but I also regained my energy and balance. What makes this treatment so helpful for me is that it fits with my lifestyle. It helps me manage my weight and energy levels in a more stable, consistent way.

In my twenties, I could just diet and work out to see quick results. But as I've gotten older, my body responds differently—and this has been an incredible support system for my health. GLP-1 medication has truly changed the way I care for myself, and I'm grateful for the stability and vitality it's brought back into my life.

Titrating Your Dose Down

When you started your GLP-1 journey, you gradually increased your dose in small, steady increments. Now that you've reached your goal, you'll reverse that process—reducing your dose just as gradually.

Most of my patients start maintenance by finding the lowest effective dose that still suppresses appetite enough for them to maintain their weight without causing further fat loss. Unless you achieve your fat loss goals using the lowest available dose (which does happen for some people), you're likely on a mid or high dose that you'll now start to taper down.

For most patients, dose reductions happen every eight to twelve weeks. Some may decrease their dose faster, especially if they're still losing weight or have maintained strong muscle mass. Others may take longer, especially if their appetite rebounds quickly or they need more time to stabilize at each dosage level.

Here's a sample trajectory: If you reached your goal on 15 milligrams of tirzepatide, you might step down in 2.5-milligram increments until you find your lowest effective dose for maintenance. Your dose will drop to 12.5 milligrams, then 10 milligrams, then 7.5 milligrams, and so on.

Gradually tapering down your dose is partly to help you avoid physical side effects, but it also gives you time to adapt your mindset and habits around food to the lower dosage. A slower tapering process allows you to become more accustomed to playing a more active role in appetite regulation and behavior change. Remember, your behavior, your routines, and your relationship with food are transitioning just as much as your body is. You want to be able to feel hunger again—but not all at once. Dropping your dose too quickly means that your appetite may return in a flood, which can feel overwhelming. If your appetite has been consistently at 2 or 3 on a 10-point scale, jumping to 10 overnight will make you feel ravenous. Gradually tapering down lets your body and brain recalibrate more slowly.

And if it turns out that you need a slightly higher dose to stay where you are? That's okay. Remember, the goal isn't to get off medication at all costs; it's to give you the best possible support for sustainable health.

How do you know if you're ready to lower your dose or if you might need to stay where you are for now? Signs that you may be ready to step down include:
- Your weight has been stable for at least a few months.
- Your appetite feels predictable and manageable.
- You're consistently hitting your goals for protein and strength training.

On the other hand, you might need to pause your tapering process or even temporarily increase your dose if:
- You're starting to feel hungrier than usual.
- You're struggling with food decisions.
- You're noticing signs of fat regain, especially around the waist.

Finding your maintenance dose is a dynamic process, and adjusting your medication is just another way to stay supported as your body and habits continue to evolve. As with everything else in medicine and life, finding your maintenance dose may not be linear; there may be ups and downs. The key is to continue with your doctor and follow-up appointments to create as much consistency as possible.

Factors Influencing Your Maintenance Dose

Your maintenance dose will vary from someone else's, and it depends on a few key factors: your current muscle mass, your adherence to a new lifestyle, and your economic situation. Let's take a closer look at each factor and learn how it can help shape your maintenance plan.

Your Current Muscle Mass

Muscle is your body's most metabolically active tissue, and it burns more calories at rest than fat does. The more muscle you have, the more efficiently you can maintain your goal weight, especially after fat loss.

If you finished your fat loss phase and have preserved a good amount of muscle—or better yet, gained more of it—your maintenance dose will be lower. You've built the internal support system needed to help you maintain your new weight.

If you lost a significant amount of muscle—say, more than 20 percent of your total weight loss—you may need a higher maintenance dose for now. I see this very often: Patients with the lowest amount of muscle usually require higher doses of their GLP-1 medication. It reinforces the point that muscle matters for metabolic efficiency. In this situation, a higher dose may be appropriate in the short term to prevent weight regain, but it's not a permanent solution. As you've learned, higher doses of medication often suppress appetite so strongly that it becomes difficult to consume the amount of protein you need to rebuild muscle. Without muscle, your metabolism stays less efficient. This might require you to continue a higher dose of medication for maintenance—which is not ideal. It also creates a bit of a catch-22: You need the higher dose to maintain your weight due to low muscle mass, but the dose may make it harder to rebuild that muscle. As with any other drug, lower doses are better for longer-term use.

If that's been your situation on your GLP-1 journey, don't worry—you can reverse that cycle (see "Building Muscle for Maintenance" on page 196). Once your weight has stabilized and you're ready to rebuild muscle, you may be able to lower your dose gradually—just enough for your appetite to return, making it easier to eat more protein, strength train, and slowly rebuild muscle. As your muscle mass increases, giving your metabolism a boost, you may find that you can comfortably lower your dose even further.

Your Current Relationship with Food

For many patients, GLP-1 therapy helps reset their relationship with food. Cravings diminish. Emotional eating quiets down. Meals become more intentional. By the time they reach maintenance, their behaviors have shifted enough that the medication becomes a supporting player, not the main driver of weight loss.

But not everyone reaches this point on the same timeline. Some patients find that as their dose is reduced and their appetite returns, old patterns can sneak back in, especially if muscle hasn't been rebuilt or protein intake is still low. That doesn't mean they're not trying. It just means that they need more support, and we adjust their dose accordingly and gradually. What is most important right now is noticing what's working and what isn't, and making decisions based on what your body is telling you.

Your Access to the Medication

An unfortunate truth is that GLP-1 medications are expensive. And frustratingly, the cost doesn't drop when the dose does. Whether you're taking 15 milligrams or 2.5 milligrams, the price tag is usually the same, except for Eli Lilly's direct pharmacy with the 2.5-milligram dose. Above 2.5 milligrams, the price will be similar—insurance or no insurance.

This creates a barrier for many people, and it's one I take seriously in my practice. Sometimes we adjust the frequency of injections—every other week instead of every week—to stretch a prescription further; this type of schedule is off-label. Sometimes we use samples. Sometimes we help patients find savings programs or explore alternate dosing plans that still provide coverage without driving up cost. If you're feeling stuck because of cost, talk to your prescriber. You shouldn't have to navigate this alone.

Microdosing FDA-Approved GLP-1s

If you have followed my work for a while, you might be surprised to see this sidebar. Well, I admit that my views on microdosing have evolved. I'm still skeptical about microdosing for extra health benefits, but over time, I've seen how very small "maintenance-level" doses can help certain patients hold their weight steady once active fat loss is complete. Let me explain.

Microdosing means taking a very small or "barely there" dose of a drug that would have a stronger effect at its full-strength recommended amount.

In the past, patients who reached their fat loss goal on the lowest available dose of a GLP-1 medication—let's say 2.5 milligrams of tirzepatide—had to stop their medication outright because the medication was administered in single-use, pre-filled injector pens and they didn't have any option to go lower when it came time to taper. But now, with some GLP-1s (such as brand-name Zepbound) available in vial form, patients have more flexibility with dosing. Instead of stopping outright at the lowest labeled dose, they can draw up a smaller amount.

These smaller doses allow people to ease into weight maintenance with a more tailored plan for continuing their medication. A super-responder who responded incredibly well on 2.5 milligrams and who might have successful weight maintenance with just 1.25 milligrams can now try this dosage. Patients who may do well with an even smaller dose now have the option to take just enough of a GLP-1 to provide a background level of appetite regulation while they transition fully into maintenance mode. When used thoughtfully in this situation, microdosing can be a tool to help you to maintain your weight.

You may hear or read about people who are interested in microdosing GLP-1s, not to lose weight but to enjoy the perceived "benefits" of a GLP-1. More often than not, their body composition analysis reports that they do have a high percentage of body fat and/or visceral fat with low muscle mass and, in truth, could benefit from a therapeutic dose of a GLP-1 (plus strength training).

If they have a truly healthy body composition and are still interested in microdosing for extra benefits, I tell them what I see: that they are healthy. And if they're incorporating exercise and lean protein into their lifestyle, they're already enjoying the benefits that come with a healthy body composition and don't need a GLP-1 to help them get there. Remember, skeletal muscle mass has a powerful anti-inflammatory effect when added to a decrease in visceral fat. If those two things are not present in your body composition, you likely need the regular therapeutic doses of a GLP-1, not a microdose.

A word on medical oversight: Microdosing is an off-label use of a GLP-1 medication, which means that using it in this way deviates from what is approved by the FDA. This means that microdosing requires your prescriber's close supervision. The 2024 Endocrine Society obesity-pharmacotherapy guidelines discuss tapering off GLP-1s but offer no specific recommendations on subtherapeutic microdoses. This means that providers must rely on their own clinical judgment, so many might lack expertise in this area or outright refuse to prescribe this way. If you're interested in microdosing, make sure to have this conversation with your provider early on.

Stopping Your Medication

While continuing a low dose of a GLP-1 is the most common path, some patients will stop GLP-1 treatment altogether. For some, it's a personal decision. For others, it may be medically necessary because they are planning a pregnancy or undergoing certain surgeries. Whatever the reason, it's essential that you don't stop abruptly. You don't want the process to feel as though you're flipping a switch.

Ideally, the tapering off process will follow the same gradual schedule as when you were initially increasing your dose—every eight to twelve weeks, depending on how you respond. This slow step-down helps your body and mind reacclimate to different hunger cues while giving you time to reinforce the behaviors and nutritional habits that will carry you through these changes.

If you ever need to stop your medication suddenly—whether because of insurance, cost, or a medical issue—don't panic. You still have options. The slower your weight loss was and the more consistently you've strength trained, prioritized your protein intake, and adopted sustainable habits around exercise and food, the better your odds of maintaining your weight without the medication.

In my clinical practice, patients who taper off GLP-1s most smoothly tend to share some or all of these traits.

- **Age:** These patients are often younger adults whose obesity has not been long-standing.
- **Lifestyle adaptation:** They have firmly integrated strength training and a protein-rich diet into their daily life and do not carry a strong family history of obesity (such as in my case, for example).
- **Body composition:** By the end of treatment, they have achieved true body recomposition: higher lean muscle mass and healthy levels of total and visceral fat. This

body recomposition provides a metabolic "buffer" once the drug is withdrawn, giving them a better chance of successfully staying off the medication.

That said, it's important to stay alert. If maintaining your weight off the medication starts to feel like a full-time job again—for example, if you are constantly resisting cravings or feeling mentally distracted by food—your body is giving you signs that some of your drivers of weight gain are still present. In that case, reintroducing treatment isn't a failure; it's a clinical decision to protect your health.

And remember, even if you are off medication, maintenance still requires attention and engagement. Continue tracking your protein intake, movement, and body composition—not to chase fat loss but to become aware of any changes before they become setbacks.

Lifestyle Anchors That Will Keep You Steady

Whether you stay on medication long term or eventually taper off, your lifestyle habits will always matter. Think of them as anchors, stabilizing forces that will help protect the progress you've made and reduce your reliance on outside tools over time.

Nutrition: More Flexibility, Same Priorities

As your GLP-1 dose decreases, your appetite will likely start to increase. You may find that you're eating about half a meal more per day than you were at the height of your treatment. That's okay! You're no longer aiming for a caloric deficit. The goal now is achieving caloric balance: eating roughly the same amount of fuel your body needs to function, move, and thrive without tipping the scale much in either direction.

You don't have to track every calorie to do this. Instead, pay attention to simple cues, such as your fullness as you eat, and stop eating when you're satisfied. Continue to keep protein front and center, perhaps more than ever. Protein helps preserve muscle, supports satiety, and helps you maintain a healthy body composition. Keeping your protein intake high also prevents overeating. As your appetite returns, use it as an opportunity to build protein-rich meals that will keep you strong, nourished, and satisfied.

But truly, the best way to keep track of what's happening in your body will still be regular body composition checks. Shifts in muscle mass or visceral fat will flag whether your current routine is supporting weight maintenance or not.

DON'T BE FOOLED BY "GLP-1-APPROVED" MARKETING

You may notice an influx of products labeled as "GLP-1 friendly" or "GLP-1 approved." Be cautious here; most claims are just marketing gimmicks. You don't need a branded popcorn or shake to succeed. You already know how to fuel your body.

Building Muscle for Maintenance

I've already talked about why muscle matters when you're taking a therapeutic dose of a GLP-1, but it plays just as important a role during maintenance. More muscle means greater caloric expenditure and more flexibility—in your routine, in your medication dosing, and in your overall lifestyle. If you haven't lost muscle, keep doing what you're doing! And if you gained muscle, know that I'm smiling wide as I write this. That's no small feat!

If, on the other hand, you lost some muscle along the way,

don't panic and don't label doing so as a failure. You are not a failure, and you never were. There is no better time than now to rebuild it. Return to your GPS: strength training and protein intake are your two best tools. Your strength training practice and protein intake should be consistent; I recommend continuing with the same amount of protein I recommend to each of my patients during the fat loss time frame.

Behavioral Changes: Your Progress Was Not Just Physical

While taking your GLP-1, you likely began to shift the way you think about food, movement, and self-care—and those changes are helping rewire your brain.

Every time you chose protein to nourish your body or said "No, thanks" to a third helping—not out of restriction but out of an awareness of fullness—you strengthened new neural pathways. Small decisions, repeated consistently, have reshaped your habits and your internal dialogue.

These decisions are what will help you stay consistent with your new habits. Your progress is not just a result of the medication. You've been building a new foundation—thought by thought, meal by meal, choice by choice. Don't be discouraged if some of those habits wobble during the transition off medication or into a new maintenance routine. This phase is about reinforcement. These shifts are proof that change isn't just possible—it's already happening. And it's becoming part of who you are.

But even with strong habits in place, you don't have to go it alone. In the next section, I'll talk about what long-term follow-up looks like and how continued support can help you stay steady for the long haul.

Special Situations: Navigating What Life Throws at You During Maintenance

As with anything else in life, maintaining your weight loss will not work out perfectly. And that's okay. Life happens. You'll go on vacation, celebrate holidays, navigate stressful times, and attend family gatherings. Even people who have never struggled with their weight gain a few pounds now and then after such experiences. What matters is how you respond, not whether you're flawless.

The last thing I want is for your maintenance plan to feel as though it's taking over your entire life. Here are a few common scenarios and how to approach them with flexibility and confidence.

Holidays

Food-centered holidays can feel complicated during maintenance, especially when traditions and expectations run deep and revolve around food (for example, at Thanksgiving). Some patients prefer to avoid temptation entirely and stick closely to their routine, while others may want a little more flexibility to participate in special meals. Both approaches are valid, and there are ways to facilitate either.

In my practice, I'll help a patient adjust based on their personal preference. For someone who doesn't want to risk overindulging and losing progress, I might temporarily increase their dose during that week. For someone who wants to enjoy the holiday more freely without feeling sick afterward, we might reduce the dose or skip it altogether for that week.

Vacations

Like holidays, vacations can bring anxiety, especially if you're leaving routines and foods that help you feel stable. Some patients worry about getting sick in an unfamiliar place or feel unsure about how they'll respond to meals while away. In these cases, I often work with them to plan a temporary medication pause. Skipping your maintenance dose for a week while you're traveling can be a practical choice if your goal is to enjoy your trip without appetite suppression or digestive effects. You can resume your usual dose upon your return.

Long-Term Follow-up

When I started my obesity medicine practice six years ago, I realized something that changed the way I care for patients: Those with obesity require ongoing, long-term support just like patients with type 2 diabetes, high blood pressure, or any other chronic condition. As more of my patients with obesity reached their goals and moved into maintenance, I began seeing a shift in my own practice. Follow-ups that had once been for managing type 2 diabetes became follow-ups for obesity care. The needs were just as real and the stakes just as high.

During the fat loss phase, most of my patients see me every eight to twelve weeks. Once they are in maintenance, we can space out those visits a bit more, about once every six months. Some patients stick with the eight- to twelve-week cadence for a while; it helps them stay accountable and feel supported until they feel more comfortable with managing longer stretches of time on their own. Others are ready to stretch the time between check-ins. There's no one-size-fits-all formula. But once your weight has stabilized and you feel confident navigating maintenance, you'll need to work with your provider to determine the cadence that works best for you.

In follow-up appointments, we'll discuss any setbacks you've been facing or reinforce what's working well already. We'll perform a body composition analysis (as well as any blood work that may be needed), and, based on the results of the body composition, we may discuss adjusting your dose further. You can find a checklist for follow-up appointments on page 250.

Whatever timing you choose, what matters most is that the support doesn't just drop off. You've worked hard to get here. And you deserve the care and tools to stay here.

WHEN TO BOOK AN EARLIER MAINTENANCE VISIT

Most patients check in with their providers every six months during maintenance, but you will want to call sooner if:

- The lower dose of your medication no longer tames your appetite, and small, balanced meals feel impossible.
- You notice new fat accumulation, especially around the waist, or your body composition scans show rising visceral fat.

A quick dose or lifestyle tweak now can prevent a far bigger setback down the line.

When Weight Comes Back—and What to Do About It

For many of my patients, the biggest fear after weight loss is gaining it back. When something has finally worked after years of struggle, even the thought of backsliding can feel overwhelming—especially if your past experiences of weight gain have been associated with feelings of failure on past diets or fitness plans. Let me reassure you: This is a valid feeling and incredibly common.

When Is a Weight Change Worth Flagging?

Not every fluctuation is a sign of trouble; day-to-day changes are part of normal physiology. So what's the difference between normal fluctuation and a true need to recalibrate your medication dosage? Watch for weight changes that steadily increase over several weeks—not just a spike here and there. Other signs might include appetite or cravings returning more strongly than before, clothing fitting differently in a way that feels consistent, energy dips or physical symptoms that had previously resolved, or emotional shifts, such as being more reactive around food. But the best way to stay aware of patterns over time? You guessed it: regular body composition analysis.

The Most Common Pattern Behind Weight Regain

In general, as long as you stay on your medication, stay engaged in your care, and keep an eye on changes in your body, significant regain is very unlikely—and if anything starts to shift, you'll be in a strong position to respond.

When it does happen, it usually follows a pattern. Most commonly, it's a gradual backslide that begins with a patient missing their follow-up appointments. After reaching their goal, they may believe that the journey is over. They feel ready to go it alone and assume that they no longer need to continue their medication or schedule follow-up visits. I understand the temptation to go down this path—but without ongoing support, even small changes in your habits or physiology can build on one another and lead to weight regain. Because the process is gradual, weight gain can go unnoticed until it suddenly feels like a setback.

In nearly every one of these cases, the patient who stopped taking GLP-1s eventually returns—frustrated, confused, and often blaming themselves. When they do come back, their biggest fear is: *What if the medication doesn't work this time?* I want to reassure you: That fear is common but rarely warranted. In my experience, most patients who restart treatment respond just as well the second time around. Your body still knows how to work with the tools you used before. Don't be hard on yourself if this happens. You're not starting over, you're reengaging—this time, with even more experience and deeper personal understanding.

You've Made It; Now Keep Going

Reaching your goal isn't the end of the road; it's the beginning of something new. You've spent months learning to trust yourself, rebuilding your relationship with food, and getting to know your body in an entirely new way. That work will continue in maintenance, but rather than repeating what you did in the earlier parts of your journey, you will move forward to a more empowered phase of care in which you are equipped with the right tools and support by your provider. Maybe you'll continue medication. Maybe you'll taper off. Either way, you now have a plan—and a new level of clarity—about what it takes to keep going and live your new definition of success.

In chapter 9, we'll explore what life looks like *after* GLP-1s, not just in terms of medication or weight maintenance but as a whole person stepping into a new chapter of life. Only now in this new age of obesity medicine are we beginning to understand what life looks like after that transformation. What challenges arise? What freedoms unfold? How do patients redefine their identity and health once the struggle to lose weight isn't front and center?

CHAPTER 9

After the Transformation: Facing Yourself and the World

Welcome to the new frontier. With the help of GLP-1 medications, large numbers of people are losing weight and maintaining meaningful fat loss for the first time in history—but few are prepared for what comes next. The physical transformation may be clearly visible and easy to celebrate, but the internal journey can be far less clear. And as common as this experience is becoming, we're still learning what comes after. There's no clear map—just a growing number of people figuring it out as they go.

In my experience, life after weight loss is rarely as simple and straightforward as people imagine. Yes, you've reached the goal that you set at the start of this journey, but now you're navigating something new: a world that feels both promising and disorienting. Your relationships may shift, your emotions may surprise you—and the sense of triumph you expected may be tangled with something more complicated.

You may not feel like yourself yet—or you may feel like a new version of yourself that you haven't quite come to know. Mixed emotions of pride, confusion, maybe vulnerability and sadness are more common than you might think. You're not alone in this stage, even if it sometimes feels that way.

In this chapter, we'll walk through the emotional, psychological, and social adjustments that so often follow the physical transformation caused by GLP-1 medications. I draw from the experiences of some of the greatest teachers I've had: my patients. The stories they share in my office have shown me that while weight loss is the visible milestone, the real work (and insight) often comes after.

Physical Adjustments

For many patients, the physical changes that come with weight loss are the first to happen—and often the easiest to celebrate. Clothes fit better, walking feels lighter, and joints ache less. Everyday tasks may even feel easier, maybe due to improved breathing or reduced pain. But not all the changes are so straightforward or positive. Some physical changes that patients report can be surprising, frustrating, or even a little unsettling. In this section, we'll explore some of the most common ones, and I'll offer guidance on how best to navigate them.

A Sensation of Feeling Cold

Many people who experience significant fat loss while undergoing GLP-1 therapy report an unexpected side effect: feeling cold all the time, even in mild or previously comfortable room temperatures.

Why does this happen? Fat doesn't just store energy; it also serves as insulation, helping regulate your internal temperature.

When your body fat decreases, your natural buffer against cooler temperatures does, too. Most patients with obesity are intolerant to heat or feel that they "run hot" most of the time, and those who have always felt overheated usually welcome this shift. But for others, the cold sensitivity can be truly uncomfortable and foreign—so much so that some patients think it's a sign of a health problem. While cold sensitivity is common after significant weight loss, it's not something you just have to live with. Here are some recommendations on how to minimize this sensation.

1. **Follow your GPS.**

    The two most important things you can do are (1) focus on building muscle, and (2) prioritize protein-dense foods—things you're already doing if you've been following the advice in this book. Muscle generates heat during activity and at rest, and strength training and increasing lean muscle mass can help raise your basal body temperature over time. To best support muscle growth, ensure that you consume enough protein to support your muscle mass and metabolic rate.

2. **Address your hormonal health.**

    Significant fat loss can impact hormones that play roles in body temperature regulation. Ask your doctor to check your thyroid function and sex hormones, especially if you are a woman in midlife.

3. **Dress in layers and stay active.**

    Keep layers handy, especially for extremities. Frequent light movement throughout the day helps your body circulate blood and generate body heat.

4. **Monitor for red flags.**

   If your cold sensitivity is extreme, persistent, or associated with other symptoms such as fatigue, hair thinning, or constipation, talk to your provider. These may be signs of hypothyroidism, iron-deficiency anemia, or other hormonal abnormalities.

Excess Skin

Excess skin is another common physical effect of major weight loss, but unlike cold sensitivity, it can be an emotionally charged one. Patients who lose a significant amount of weight, especially if they had severe obesity, often have excess skin that doesn't retract fully. This can cause discomfort, impact confidence, and even lead to medical complications such as skin irritation or infections.

If excess skin is a concern for you, I encourage you to consult with a qualified plastic surgeon and explore the possibility of skin removal surgery. It is important to look for a doctor who does this type of surgery often.

For some people, the choice to undergo surgery is about comfort or medical necessity, such as skin irritation or mobility issues. For others, it's about feeling more confident and at home in their body. Both reasons are valid.

If surgery is not something you can—or want to—pursue, here are some recommendations to help you manage excess skin.

- **Be patient; skin remodeling takes time.** Skin can continue to tighten gradually for twelve to twenty-four months after weight loss. Younger patients and those with higher collagen and elastin levels may see more natural retraction.

- **Build muscle volume to improve your skin's appearance.** Sound familiar? Yes, there is one more reason to focus on muscle. Resistance training can fill out loose areas by increasing muscle mass underneath the skin. Focus on compound lifts (squats, deadlifts, rows) to promote full-body toning and strengthening. Muscle adds structure, improves appearance, and helps prevent further sagging.
- **Support your skin health from within.** Ensure that your protein intake is sufficient to support collagen synthesis and skin integrity. Nutrients important for elasticity include vitamin C, zinc, and omega-3 fatty acids. Hydration is important, too.
- **Explore treatment options, if desired.** If your excess skin is causing rashes, mobility difficulties, or psychological distress, there are treatment options available, both surgical and nonsurgical. Surgical treatments such as body contouring procedures (panniculectomy, brachioplasty, and others) are typically recommended after significant weight loss and once your weight has been stable for six to twelve months. Nonsurgical options may help improve skin texture and tightness after more moderate weight loss. These include radio frequency or ultrasound therapy, microneedling with PRP, and prescription-strength topical retinoids.

Loss of Facial Volume (aka "Ozempic Face")

The term "Ozempic face" has made headlines. (I was even quoted in a *New York Times* article about it!) But while the name is new, the phenomenon of facial volume loss isn't. What people are noticing is a common and natural part of significant weight loss—especially when fat is lost from the face.

For some people, loss of fat creates a more sculpted or angular appearance. For others, the change can be more dramatic. Facial volume loss tends to show up most in the cheeks, temples, and under-eye area and is often more pronounced in individuals who lose weight rapidly or have lower baseline body fat to begin with. Again, this isn't just about an aesthetic concern, and it also provides an example of why nutritional support is important during any weight loss journey. If your protein intake is inadequate during the fat-loss process, you are more likely to experience loss of facial volume because inadequate protein leads to a decline in the production of collagen and elastin, two key components of your skin that help maintain its structure, elasticity, and volume. As a result, your skin may appear looser, thinner, or more aged.

Getting enough protein and losing weight at a gradual pace are both key to minimizing this unwanted side effect. Even then, there can be some volume loss. If you're struggling with these changes, you do have options. A consultation with a qualified provider—whether for skin support as discussed in the "excess skin" section above or other nonsurgical treatments—can help you feel more comfortable with your appearance and understand your options.

Changes in Foot Size and Shoe Fit

It might surprise you to learn that weight loss can change your feet. When you carry excess weight, your feet bear that load every day. Over time, this extra pressure can flatten the arches (leading to wider or longer feet), increase the fat padding in the soles and tops of the feet, and cause foot and ankle swelling, making your shoes feel tight. After significant weight loss, these changes may begin to reverse. You might notice that your feet feel different and function differently. You may even need to wear a different shoe size. To help your feet adjust, here's what I recommend.

- **Remeasure your feet.** You may need a different shoe size or width.
- **Find shoes with support or consider inserts.** With less fat padding, cushioning and arch support become more important.
- **Consult a podiatrist.** This is especially important if you experience new foot pain or instability or need orthotic guidance.
- **Be patient.** Just like the rest of your body, your feet are adjusting to a new normal.

Breast Changes

Breasts are composed of both glandular tissue and fat, and for many women, a significant portion of breast volume is fatty tissue. That means that when you lose weight through a method that promotes fat loss, such as GLP-1 therapy, the size, shape, volume, and firmness of your breasts might change, too. For some people, these changes are welcome. For others, they may make them feel less like themselves. While you can't control where your body loses fat, you can support the transition. Here are some suggestions for how to do so.

- **Prioritize skin and collagen health.** Prioritize adequate protein, hydration, and nutrients such as vitamin C, zinc, and omega-3s, which are crucial for skin repair and elasticity.
- **Strength train.** While it won't restore breast volume, strength training can build the pectoral muscles underneath the breasts, providing a small lift and improving overall chest appearance and posture.
- **Invest in proper bra support.** A professional bra fitting after weight loss can make a big difference in your comfort, appearance, and confidence.

- **Talk to a provider if it's affecting your mental health.** For some women, the change in breast appearance can be emotionally difficult. In those cases, discussing options such as nonsurgical skin tightening or, if appropriate, surgical lifts or reconstruction can be empowering.

Sleep Changes

Improved sleep is one of the most overlooked benefits of weight loss. For some people, it's the first time in years they've been able to sleep deeply, breathe easily, and wake up feeling refreshed. This is especially true for people who had obstructive sleep apnea before treatment. Excess fat, particularly around the neck and upper airway, can contribute to airway obstruction, so weight loss can dramatically reduce apnea symptoms.

In some cases, patients who have undergone GLP-1 therapy are able to stop using their continuous positive airway pressure (CPAP) machine, the most common treatment for sleep apnea, altogether, but of course, if you were diagnosed with sleep apnea in the past, it's important to talk to your provider before discontinuing or making any changes to your treatment.

In other cases, sleep may temporarily get worse before it gets better. During periods of rapid weight loss, changes in hormones, blood sugar, or medication timing can make it harder to fall or stay asleep. Some patients report light sleep, vivid dreams, or restlessness. And for many, sleep disruption has nothing to do with physiology at all and instead reflects the emotional impact of these changes. If you're struggling with sleep, here are tips that can help.

- **Create a consistent wind-down routine.** This is especially helpful during periods of hormonal adjustment, which occur as your body adapts to fat loss or medication changes.

- **Monitor your sleep hygiene.** Limit screen time before bed, keep your room at a comfortable temperature and dark, and establish regular sleep/wake times.
- **Don't underestimate emotional factors.** Journaling, therapy, or support groups can help manage the psychological impact of the physical changes caused by GLP-1s.
- **Talk to your provider if your sleep changes persist.** If your sleep doesn't improve, especially if you've stopped CPAP after weight loss or notice lingering fatigue, it may be time to reassess your sleep apnea or check your labs.

Psychological Adjustments

When people think about weight loss, they often picture the physical results: new clothing sizes, before-and-after photos, maybe compliments from others. But the emotional impact can run much deeper and feel less predictable.

In this section, we'll explore the emotional shifts that may follow significant weight loss. Even when the weight loss is intentional, healthy, and empowering, many patients are surprised by how complicated it can feel to live in a body that's now different. Reaching a long-held goal doesn't always bring immediate clarity and confidence; in fact, it can cause confusion, disorientation, or even grief. Some patients are caught completely off guard by their own reactions. I've found this to be one of the most fascinating—and humbling—parts of practicing obesity medicine. With each patient, I've learned that behind every weight loss goal, there is a whole person with hopes, fears, and a lifetime of experiences shaped by their body. As doctors, we're trained to treat a disease—but watching the journey of each of my patients reminds me to treat the person.

Shifting Your Self-Perception

After years, sometimes decades, of believing that meaningful weight loss was out of reach, you arrive at a new, healthy weight, yet your mind may struggle to catch up. The transformation is real and the metrics show it, but internally, it may still feel as though your previous body still lingers. You look at your reflection and sometimes can't fully absorb or accept the change.

Many of my patients express similar feelings. They tell me, "I see myself in the mirror, but I don't recognize who that person is," or "I don't feel like I can celebrate—it still feels like the rug is about to get pulled out from under me."

Years spent living with a body carrying excess weight—a body that is deeply tied to how you see yourself—means that your self-image may not change at the same speed as the physical changes that you saw while on GLP-1 treatment. That lag can create anxiety. Compliments about your progress might feel awkward, and you might not be sure exactly how to receive them. When I see this disconnect happening in my patients, I try to bring them back to one simple truth: Transformation isn't just physical; your brain and emotions are still catching up. Give them time to process.

Reconciling Your Relationship with Your Body

While your body's transformation is measurable and visible, it doesn't automatically erase the emotional scars caused by years of being treated differently or the feelings of unworthiness that stem from a lifetime of that treatment. For many patients, the way others treated them before weight loss—whether through bias, rejection, or exclusion—left wounds that don't disappear just because their body has changed. And sometimes these unhealed experiences resurface even more strongly once the weight is gone.

Some of my patients, anticipating this, begin therapy even *be-*

fore starting their weight loss treatment, knowing that it may help them sort through these feelings before the physical changes come in and muddy the waters. Doing that work—unlearning old messages, rebuilding self-worth, addressing years of stigma or shame—is just as important as changing your eating habits or medication dose.

It's okay to have contradictory feelings about reaching your goal weight. It's okay if your joy is mixed with disbelief and part of you is waiting for the other shoe to drop. When those difficult feelings start to surface—if old insecurities, trauma, or questions about self-worth begin to come up, understand that they are part of the healing process.

Healing your body and healing your relationship with your body are two separate journeys. Both take time, self-compassion, and sometimes professional support. If difficult feelings are starting to surface, consider talking to a therapist. Just as your medical team supported your physical progress, a mental health professional can help you navigate the emotional side of what comes next. Acknowledge that the internal work is as essential as the physical changes—and that emotional reactions can be complex, even when things are going well.

Social Adjustments

Your internal experience can be intense; your *external* experience—how others react to the "new" you—can be, too. And just like your emotions, other people's responses to your physical changes may surprise you.

You might expect your loved ones to be thrilled for you. And many of them will be! But some reactions can feel . . . off or not what you expected. They may be muted, confusing, even hurtful.

Some patients tell me that people around them aren't as happy as they'd expected. You may hear comments such as "You're too skinny!" or "Stop losing weight—you don't look like yourself anymore."

Handling Negative Comments

Many people with obesity or overweight have people close to them who struggle with their own weight. They may have their own complicated relationship with food, body image, or control or simply feel unprepared for how much you've changed. Often, their comments come from a place of discomfort, not malice. The people who are saying them may be adjusting to the changes that they see in you. Their reactions reflect their own insecurities more than anything else.

You should continue to feel proud—not just for the physical changes you've accomplished but for the strength and resilience it takes to achieve and maintain them. Understand that some people may comment on your appearance without understanding or seeing the invisible victories: stabilized blood sugar, regulated hunger cues, better sleep, clearer thinking, quieted shame. They may not recognize the emotional weight you've shed, the habits you've rewired, or the courage it took to ask for help in the first place. And while their discomfort, skepticism, or unsolicited opinions may be hurtful, they do not diminish your choices.

Still, even when you intellectually know that awkward comments will be made, they may not be easy to navigate in the moment. Whether you're dealing with nosy questions, backhanded compliments, or well-meaning but off-putting praise, it can help to think ahead of time about how you'll respond.

QUICK SCRIPTS FOR SOCIAL SITUATIONS

Sometimes it's not a big deal for someone to make a comment about your weight loss. Other times, it can feel uncomfortable and invasive. Remember that you don't owe anyone an explanation or have to stay in a conversation that makes you feel uncomfortable. Here are some short, simple responses that can help you maintain your boundaries, redirect the conversation, or shut it down.

If you want to acknowledge the comment but shift the focus:
- "Thanks—I'm focusing on my health these days."
- "I'm feeling better, and that's what matters most!"

If you want to shut down intrusive or judgmental questions:
- "That's a really personal topic, and I'd rather not get into it."
- "Yeah, I've found something that's working for me. Did you watch the new episode of _____ yet?"

If someone makes a backhanded compliment or seems uncomfortable with your progress:
- "I know change can be a lot to process—it is for me, too."
- "I feel good about where I'm at. I hope you can support that."

If you want to be direct and move on:
- "I'm happy and feeling good. That's enough for me!"
- "But enough talking about me. How are you doing?"

Confronting Weight Stigma

Weight stigma is real—and unfortunately, it's deeply embedded in our society and culture. If you've struggled with your weight for a long time, you've likely experienced it firsthand: the bias, the judgment, the subtle (or not-so-subtle) ways people treat you differently because of your body. Over time, you may have come to expect it. You may have even internalized it. And that's heartbreaking; no one should ever have to accept mistreatment like this as normal.

What many people who experience significant weight loss aren't prepared for is how easy it is to see the signs of weight stigma all around them. You might notice people suddenly being . . . nicer. More complimentary or respectful. Holding the door and making eye contact. Asking questions they never would have asked you before. And while some of that may feel validating, it can also stir up complex emotions: grief, anger, confusion, and even resentment. Because now you're seeing weight stigma from a new vantage point. You weren't imagining it. You're now witnessing firsthand how differently the world responds to different bodies—and realizing how unjust that difference is from this new perspective can be absolutely *crushing*.

If this resonates with you, please know that you're not alone. You don't have to sort through those feelings on your own. This is another area where I strongly encourage you to talk to a psychotherapist or mental health professional to help you process these shifts, especially if they bring up old wounds or make you question your worth. I would encourage you to look for support groups in your area or even on social media.

It's also common to find yourself, perhaps unexpectedly, experiencing bias in the opposite direction: You may catch yourself judging someone else's eating habits or thinking critically about another person's body in a way you wouldn't have before. If you have these thoughts, they don't make you a bad person; they reflect the same weight stigma you were subjected to, and they prove just how pervasive it is. Respond to these thoughts with awareness, not shame. When you notice them come up, meet them with curiosity and compassion—not just for others but for yourself. Give yourself grace. Your transformation, both inside and out, is ongoing.

And as you move through emotions, please remember that not everyone has access to the same life-changing tools that you do. Be proud of your progress, but stay grounded in empathy. Wouldn't it be amazing if GLP-1 medications didn't just change bodies but also helped us change the way we empathize with and accept all bodies?

Sharing Your Journey

For most patients, sharing their GLP-1 journey is a deeply personal decision. Some patients are open from day one and want to share their experiences with the world. Others tell no one, not even their spouse. There's no single right way to approach what to communicate with others, and I fully respect every person's choice.

But if you're keeping your use of GLP-1 medication private because you are worried people will judge you or accuse you of taking the easy way out, I invite you to consider another point of view. When patients choose not to tell others about their GLP-1 treatment, it can unintentionally reinforce the harmful myth that weight loss is purely a matter of willpower. Someone close to you, who's watched you struggle for years, may see your progress and think, "She did it on her own. Why can't I?" And just like that, the misconceptions about obesity live on.

That's why when you feel safe and ready, I encourage you to share your story, especially with those who love you. Your openness has the potential to shift not just your personal relationships but also an *entire cultural conversation*. If we want to normalize obesity treatment as legitimate medical care, it has to start with those of us who have used GLP-1 therapy telling our stories and describing our experiences. Being transparent with people you trust can not only bring you closer to them but also open the door to support—something you need as you maintain your progress. Think about social situations such as dinners or celebrations:

You'll want the people around you to understand your reality and not push food on you, comment on your portions, or encourage you to have a drink you're not interested in. That kind of support is easier to come by when people can see the full picture instead of trying to piece things together for themselves.

Most of the time, people will be grateful for your honesty and vulnerability. People who care for you and value your happiness and health will make their support clear to you. You might also find out who may not have your best interests at heart—and that's important information to unearth, too.

So the next time you are hesitant to share your story, ask yourself: **What is keeping me from feeling comfortable with sharing my story?** Could your hesitancy be rooted in shame—or even your own anti-obesity bias? Deep down, are you one of those people who still thinks that taking weight loss medications is "cheating" or "taking the easy way out"? Let me say this again: If you followed the guidance in this book, your weight loss wasn't easy; it took real effort and dedication. This time your effort paid off because you finally had the medical support your body needed to succeed. And this is a message that is worth sharing with others.

CASSIE'S STORY

I've struggled with my weight and body image for as long as I can remember. My weight fluctuated throughout my life, into my thirties. I've always been athletic—I love skiing, running, and yoga—but despite my active lifestyle, it felt impossible to reach and maintain the weight I wanted to be.

By the time I found Dr. Salas-Whalen, I was in a deep depression and at my heaviest weight: 230 pounds. I had been scared to step on the scale for years. Seeing that number filled me with so much shame and hopelessness that I began to abuse substances to cope. I've struggled with impulse control for as long as I can remember, and it felt like everything was unraveling. When I was referred to Dr. Salas-Whalen, I had no idea how life changing GLP-1 treatment was going to be.

I started a GLP-1 medication and made a commitment to myself to live an active and healthy lifestyle. I began practicing hot yoga and eating a Mediterranean diet. In the first month on GLP-1, I lost seven pounds, which motivated me to keep going. For the first time in a long time, I felt encouraged. I felt confident enough to start dating again. I liked how I looked and felt in clothes. I started to enjoy shopping again. Slowly, the feeling of shame was beginning to lift. I started to love and feel proud of myself. I was happy again.

Eventually, I lost a total of 100 pounds. But the physical transformation wasn't the most profound part. My cravings for substances and emotional eating dissipated. I couldn't believe it! My thinking started to change, and I achieved a full year of sobriety.

GLP-1 medication—and the support of Dr. Salas-Whalen—didn't just impact my life on a physical level; they helped me build a life I'd never thought that I could have. They gave me the ability to create the change that I have been wanting and working hard toward my entire life. For that, I am forever grateful.

Living in the "After"

Reaching your goal weight may have once felt like the finish line—the solution to everything, the moment when life would finally begin. Maybe you pictured it like the second frame in a before-and-after photo: a glossier, healthier, happier you. Now that you're here, you may be realizing something no one talks about enough: that life after GLP-1 therapy brings its own set of physical, emotional, and social adjustments that are just as complex as the weight loss itself.

You've shed more than just pounds; you may have also let go of shame, self-doubt, and the old beliefs that told you that you weren't trying hard enough. You've built new habits, practiced discipline, made sacrifices, and learned to advocate for your health. That deserves to be honored, but reaching this point doesn't mean that every struggle will disappear. You may still have days when your body feels unfamiliar or when your mind is catching up to the changes you see in the mirror. You may still feel surprised by the way others treat you differently or by the unexpected grief for the version of you that carried all that weight—physically and emotionally—for so long. This is the real work of transformation. It doesn't end at a number on the scale. It lives in the quiet, complicated moments that follow: in the relationships you rebuild, in the confidence you rediscover, in the way you learn to live fully—without waiting for "someday."

But don't mistake the road ahead as a setback; this is a new beginning. All the space that the food noise and the weight loss wishes used to occupy is *yours* now, and you get to decide what to fill it with.

What's next on your list of things you once thought were impossible? Maybe a new job? A career pivot? A solo trip you've been quietly imagining for years? What would be the smallest first step toward that goal? Could you take it today? I want you to begin imagining a life beyond the struggle to lose weight, because that chapter is behind you now. You've done something extraordinary: You've learned to work with your body using new tools, new understanding, and a belief that lasting change is possible.

The "after" isn't theoretical anymore; it's you. You're no longer imagining who you could be, because you already *are*. You've been here all along. The only thing left is to live like it: stronger, freer, and more in tune with yourself. The next chapter is yours to write. Before I leave you to create it, I'll share a few final reflections to carry with you as you move into it.

A Final Word

For years, I've wanted to write a book about obesity and GLP-1 medications because there was a message that the world urgently needed to hear—something that each of my patients has shown me: that we've misunderstood obesity and we've deeply misjudged the people living with it.

What I discovered was this: No one wants to lose excess weight more than the person who is struggling to carry it, not just to feel healthier but to feel at home in their body. To feel free. I hope this book has shown you how a medical tool can make that dream of freedom a reality. This freedom doesn't mean stepping back from managing your own health and letting a medication take over. It's about stepping forward, finally able to engage with your health in a way that is realistic. When the barriers that have kept you stuck begin to fall away, your ability to participate in your own care will change. You will realize that you are capable—and that your body *can* be responsive. It can be a partner in your health, not an adversary.

I know I've said it many times: GLP-1s require work. But what starts as work settles into something different. It becomes rhythm—health maintenance that feels so good that it is rewarding in and of itself. And soon it feels like *peace*—a well-earned, deeply personal sense of peace.

For so many people who use a GLP-1 medication, the battle with food and weight was all-consuming. For some, that battle meant living in a body that was unresponsive, judged, and misunderstood. For others, it meant clawing their way to an "acceptable" weight—appearing "fine" on the outside but white-knuckling every meal, every decision, every craving. Both ways of living were exhausting, physically, mentally, and emotionally.

I hope that this book—and treatment—brings you relief. Relief from the weight of constant mental noise and shame and from the endless loop of restriction and rebound. I hope that you are able to think clearly, eat intentionally, move freely—perhaps for the first time. I hope that you no longer battle your body but begin to work with it.

And while this book is written for anyone walking this path, I also hope it speaks to the people who care for them: family members, friends, even fellow clinicians who want to understand. If you're here not for yourself but for someone you love (or treat), I hope that this book has deepened your empathy.

GLP-1 medications don't just offer personal breakthroughs. They have also jump-started cultural and medical shifts. They have already proven to be groundbreaking, but I believe we're still at the very beginning of their impact. As these medications become more widely understood and responsibly used, we'll see effects far beyond the individual scale.

I predict that we'll see many positive changes in the years ahead (you read about them here first!):

- People will live longer lives with a better quality of life.
- More people will be fit and strong. They will find it easier to stick with workout plans, and we might see more people in the gym.
- There will be less alcohol consumption.

And for the generations ahead, we might see:
- Declines in chronic diseases, including type 2 diabetes
- A stronger, healthier military and police force, making our communities safer
- A decline in the incidence of obesity-linked cancers (colon, pancreatic, prostate, and others)
- Some medical specialties that currently treat the complications of obesity are shrinking or disappearing altogether
- Evolution in the food industry, which will be forced to offer products that align with how people actually want to feel in their bodies

I can't think of a more powerful note to end on than this. GLP-1 medications do more than promise progress in the treatment of obesity; they have the power to dismantle the very factors that created the obesity epidemic in the first place. A food landscape that once profited from addictive, highly processed products will begin to lose its grip. These environmental, cultural, and even biological shifts have the potential to loosen obesity's hold on the future.

Maybe this isn't just the beginning of a new era of obesity treatment; maybe it's the beginning of a new era of good health.

In the meantime, my hope is that something in this book will help you see GLP-1 therapy through clear eyes. Yes, I wrote this book because I want the science on GLP-1 therapy to be better understood. I want patients to feel empowered and informed and to navigate their treatment journey safely. I want doctors to change the way they approach treatment. But more than that, I hope that the experiences I've shared will help all of us relate differently to ourselves and to one another. Maybe you've recognized yourself or someone you love in these pages. Maybe reading this book will change the way you interpret a stranger's body on an airplane. Maybe it will help you extend more grace—both to others and to yourself.

That's how change begins. At its core, this book isn't just about shedding physical weight; it's about releasing the shame that was never yours to carry, the guilt that dimmed your joy, and the restrictions that kept you small. My deepest wish for you is this: that you become truly **weightless**—unburdened, empowered, and free.

PROTEIN CHEAT SHEET

Your Protein Game Plan

To help you manage your protein intake, here is a protein game plan with six simple guidelines to follow.

1. **Aim to consume 100+ grams of protein per day.** To preserve muscle while losing weight, you need enough total protein if you're on a GLP-1. That means at least 100 grams a day—minimum!

2. **Start early.** Getting a solid dose of protein within the first hour or so of waking up gives you a head start and helps distribute your intake across the day, which is much easier on your appetite than trying to cram it all in at the end. If you're someone who puts creamer or milk into your coffee, add a scoop of unflavored or flavored whey protein instead.

3. **Count no more than 30 grams of protein per meal.** Aim to space your protein in about four portions of around 25 grams of protein, but tally no more than 30 grams of protein at a time in your daily total. Your body can use only so much protein at once to build or preserve muscle. Research shows that 30 grams is about the maximum amount of protein your body will direct toward muscle preservation/development at any given meal (anything above the 30 grams per meal is not wasted; it goes to support other bodily functions).

4. **Give your body time between meals.** Space your meals at least three to four hours apart. Protein is very filling; if you don't allow enough time between supplementation and meals, you won't be able to consume the amount of protein you need in a day.

5. **Get the protein off your plate first.** This will ensure that you meet your target protein intake even if your appetite dips midway through your meal.

6. **Drink protein shakes.** Protein shakes and powders are a great way to supplement. Many patients are successful with keeping to a roughly fifty/fifty ratio of protein shakes and meals—this ensures that you have a quick and easy way to load up on protein but don't end up feeling undernourished or experience low energy from lack of food. As you plan your day, remember not to have any shakes too close to meals; you don't want a shake making you feel full when it's time to eat!

What Does 30 Grams of Protein Look Like?

Meat and Poultry
- 4 ounces (113 grams) cooked chicken breast
- 4 ounces (113 grams) cooked lean ground beef or ground turkey
- 5 ounces (140 grams) cooked turkey breast
- 5 ounces (140 grams) cooked pork loin
- 4 slices turkey bacon (only if high protein, about 7–8 grams per slice)

Fish and Seafood
- 5 ounces (140 grams) cooked salmon
- 5–6 ounces (140–170 grams) canned tuna in water
- 6 ounces (170 grams) cooked shrimp
- 6 ounces (170 grams) cooked cod or tilapia

Dairy and Eggs
- 1¼ cups cottage cheese
- 1½ cups Greek yogurt
- 5 large eggs
- 1½ cups egg whites (approximately 12)

Vegetarian Proteins and Legumes
- ¾ cup (about 150 grams) firm tofu
- 2 cups cooked lentils or chickpeas
- 3¾ cups cooked quinoa

Pantry Staples
- 1 scoop (30–35 grams) whey isolate protein powder
- 3 cups bone broth (only if high protein, about 10 grams per cup)
- 1¾ cups high-protein pasta (e.g., chickpea, lentil, or edamame based)

FIRST APPOINTMENT CHECKLIST

Use this checklist to help you prepare for your first appointment. Your provider will want to understand your full medical history and personal context in order to tailor your treatment plan.

Bring or Be Prepared to Discuss

1. **Your personal weight history**
   - Your age when weight changes began
   - Your past efforts to manage your weight
   - What has or hasn't worked

2. **Your family weight and health history**
   - Family members with obesity, diabetes, thyroid disorders, PCOS, or heart disease

3. **Your current health status**
   - Your medical diagnoses
   - Your current medications and supplements
   - Your known allergies or sensitivities

4. **Your diet and eating habits**
   - Your typical meals and snacks
   - Any regularly occurring night eating, binge eating, and/or emotional eating
   - Your use of meal replacements or specialty diets

5. **Your exercise and activity levels**
   - Your weekly activity (type, frequency, duration)
   - Any physical limitations or injuries

6. **Your hormone and menstrual history (if applicable)**
   - Your menstrual cycle regularity or irregularity

- Your history of polycystic ovarian syndrome (PCOS), perimenopause, menopause, or use of hormone-replacement therapy (HRT)

7. **Your mental and emotional health**
   - Your history of depression, anxiety, ADHD, or trauma
   - Your stress level and coping mechanisms

8. **Your relationship with food and your body**
   - Your history of eating disorders or disordered eating
   - Your current mindset regarding food, weight, and control

9. **Your social and environmental context**
   - Your support system at home and/or work
   - Your lifestyle constraints (e.g., frequent travel, caregiving, shift work)

10. **Your alcohol, tobacco, or substance use**

Questions to Ask

- What do I need to know about my access to medications, insurance coverage, and brand-name versus compounded medications?
- Will my body composition be assessed, and how?
- What labs may be ordered (e.g., A1C, TSH, cholesterol, liver enzymes)?
- What will happen after this appointment?
- How often will I be seen?
- Will I receive a prescription for my first dose today?
- What dose will I start at?
- What will happen if I don't tolerate the medication well?
- What support is available between appointments?

FOLLOW-UP APPOINTMENT CHECKLIST

Follow-up visits are essential for evaluating how you're responding to treatment and what type of support you may need, as well as for making dose adjustments.

Bring or Be Prepared to Discuss

1. **Changes in your appetite or cravings**
   - Has your hunger decreased, stayed the same, or returned?
   - Are you experiencing food aversions or nausea?

2. **Changes in your weight and body composition**
   - Are there any changes in your weight or how your clothes fit?
   - If applicable, review data from your at-home scale.

3. **Changes in your protein intake**
   - Are you meeting your daily protein goal (typically 90 to 100 grams or more)?
   - Are you using shakes or supplements?
   - Are you having any difficulty consuming enough protein?

4. **Your exercise and physical activity**
   - Are you strength training regularly?
   - Has your physical activity increased, decreased, or remained steady?

5. **Your muscle mass and energy level**
   - Are you feeling weaker, stronger, or the same?
   - Do you have any signs of fatigue or low endurance?

6. **Your medication tolerance**
   - Have there been any side effects (nausea, constipation, fatigue, etc.)?

- Did you miss any doses?
- Have you made any dose adjustments on your own?

7. **Your menstrual or hormonal changes (if applicable)**

8. **Your emotional and mental health**
   - Have you experienced mood changes, brain fog, or emotional reactions to weight loss?
   - Do you have any signs of anxiety, depression, or body image issues?

9. **Your sleep quality and patterns**
   - Do you see any improvements or new difficulties?

10. **Your support and accountability**
    - Are you tracking your food intake or habits?
    - Do you have any new challenges at home or work?
    - Do you have any need for referrals (e.g., nutritionist, therapist, personal trainer)?

11. **Questions or concerns for your provider**
    - Should we change the dose?
    - When will I taper?
    - What are my current goals?
    - What do I need to focus on before the next visit?

12. **Your labs or diagnostics**
    - Review any new lab results.
    - Plan for upcoming lab work if needed.

Acknowledgments

To my daughters: Thank you for being so patient with Mommy. I am sorry I missed swimming lessons and track meets while I wrote this book. Thank you for telling Mommy "It's okay, you should write." I am so very proud of both of you. Being your mommy is the biggest gift I've received. Love my girls.

To my dad: Thank you for believing I could do anything I wanted to do. In your eyes, nothing was an impossible for me. You saw I could fly, and you let me be free. I hope you left knowing the huge impression and impact you made on my life. I miss our conversations over a cup of coffee at Sanborns.

To my mom: In my younger years, we didn't see eye to eye. We didn't understand each other; you couldn't understand why I wanted to be a doctor, to move from our hometown, to leave my country, to leave you. I am sorry I misjudged you so many times. I am sorry that at the time I didn't have the maturity to comprehend you. I am sorry you didn't have the opportunity and the time for yourself to also feel free, to learn to enjoy life without thinking of somebody else for a change. I am angry that I didn't get to enjoy you more and that you didn't get to fly, wild and free. I will wait patiently to see you again and make up for the lost time. One day, Mom, one day I won't leave you ever again.

To my brothers and sisters-in-law: Thank you for taking care of my parents after I left. Thanks to all of you, I left our home knowing our parents were well taken care of, filled with love and grandchildren. Lalo and Adrian, I love you so very much. We don't have our parents now, but we have one another.

To my dear friends Dina, Daniela, Grace: Dina, you are my sister, no doubt. Thank you for always keeping me grounded. Thank you for always being there when I've needed you the most. I still remember the exact moment we met each other. You were wearing jean overalls and a white T-shirt. You were sitting, and I was standing. It all started with my shoes. I will book our rooms at the fanciest nursing home, my friend. Together till the end.

My dear Daniela, you have also been with me since the beginning, through all my crazy and not-so-crazy decisions. Thank you for choosing our friendship above anything. I am truly grateful for you. Thank you for keeping me on a tight allowance.

My dear Grace, I wish you could see yourself as I see you. In the short time we have known each other, you have shown me so much love and grace. Thank you for believing in me and supporting me along the way.

To my dear nanny Mari: Having you in my life has allowed me to build, to work, and even to write this book. Thank you for loving my girls as much as I do, thank you for giving me a state of peace while you watch my kids. I am so proud of you! You are one strong, smart, and go-getter woman. Your sons are so proud of you.

To my New York Endocrinology team: Thank you for taking such good care of my patients and my office. Each of you contributes so much at work. Our patients love you all and always tell me how helpful you are. Thank you from the bottom of my heart. Tere, ponte a estudiar!

To my patients: I am who I am because of you. Your trust in me will never be taken for granted. I hope you know how proud I am of every single one of you. I know I tend to carry a big stick in my practice, but it's because you deserve the best possible outcome of your health. I will see you every three months!

Thank you to my book agents, Amanda and Kim, to my editor, Elysia, for always being there to answer any questions and concerns, and to the rest of my publishing team at Penguin Random House: Marnie, Theresa, Danielle, Lulu, Hannah, and Cindy.

And finally, thank you to Danielle, for helping me bring this book to life with care and conviction.

Notes

Introduction

xv **third leading cause of death:** "Mexico: Health Data Overview for the United Mexican States," World Health Organization, accessed June 6, 2025, https://data.who.int/countries/484.

Chapter 1

5 **obesity rates have nearly tripled:** W. P. T. James, "WHO Recognition of the Global Obesity Epidemic," *International Journal of Obesity* 32, suppl. 7 (2008): S120–S126, https://doi.org/10.1038/ijo.2008.247.

5 **13 percent of U.S. adults:** Cheryl D. Fryar, Margaret D. Carroll, and Joseph Afful, "Prevalence of Overweight, Obesity, and Severe Obesity Among Adults Aged 20 and Over: United States, 1960–1962 Through 2017–2018," National Center for Health Statistics, 2020, https://www.cdc.gov/nchs/data/hestat/obesity-adult-17-18/overweight-obesity-adults-H.pdf.

5 **skyrocketed to 30.5 percent:** Katherine M. Flegal et al., "Prevalence and Trends in Obesity Among US Adults, 1999–2000," *JAMA* 288, no. 14 (2002): 1723–27, https://doi.org/10.1001/jama.288.14.1723

5 **41.9 percent of U.S. adults:** "Adult Obesity Facts," Centers for Disease Control and Prevention, May 14, 2024, https://www.cdc.gov/obesity/adult-obesity-facts/index.html.

6 **nearly one in five children:** "Childhood Obesity Facts," Centers for Disease Control and Prevention, April 2, 2024, https://www.cdc.gov/obesity/childhood-obesity-facts/childhood-obesity-facts.html?CDC_AAref_Va_=https://www.cdc.gov/obesity/data/childhood.html.

6 **nearly half of U.S. adults:** Zachary J. Ward et al., "Projected U.S. State-

Level Prevalence of Adult Obesity and Severe Obesity," *New England Journal of Medicine* 381, no. 25 (2019): 2440–50, https://doi.org/10.1056/NEJMsa1909301.

6 **from the United Kingdom to China:** "Obesity and Overweight," World Health Organization, 2023, https://www.who.int/news-room/fact-sheets/detail/obesity-and-overweight.

6 **more than thirteen obesity-related cancers:** Elizabeth L. Miller and Sarah J. Thompson, "Awareness of Obesity-Related Cancers: A Complex Issue," *International Journal of Environmental Research and Public Health* 19, no. 11 (2022): 6617, https://doi.org/10.3390/ijerph19116617.

6 **it can shorten lifespan significantly:** Nicola Di Daniele et al., "Impact of Mediterranean Diet on Metabolic Syndrome, Cancer and Longevity," *Oncotarget* 8, no. 5 (2017): 8947–79, https://doi.org/10.18632/oncotarget.13553.

9 **Obesity was recognized as a disease:** James, "WHO Recognition of the Global Obesity Epidemic."

11 **Obesity is profoundly influenced:** Nadia Panera et al., "Genetics, Epigenetics and Transgenerational Transmission of Obesity in Children," *Frontiers in Endocrinology* 13 (2022): 1006008, https://doi.org/10.3389/fendo.2022.1006008.

11 **Some people are biologically predisposed:** Jennifer L. Elks et al., "Variability in the Heritability of Body Mass Index: A Systematic Review and Meta-regression," *Frontiers in Endocrinology* 3 (2012): 29, https://doi.org/10.3389/fendo.2012.00029.

11 **due to genetic inheritance and epigenetic modifications:** Ruth J. F. Loos and Giles S. H. Yeo, "The Genetics of Obesity: From Discovery to Biology," *Nature Reviews Genetics* 23, no. 2 (2022): 120–33, https://doi.org/10.1038/s41576-021-00414-z.

11 **If you have a family history:** Cheng Huang, Wei Chen, and Xiaojun Wang, "Studies on the Fat Mass and Obesity-Associated (FTO) Gene and Its Impact on Obesity-Associated Diseases," *Genes & Diseases* 10, no. 6 (2022): 2351–65, https://doi.org/10.1016/j.gendis.2022.04.014.

11 **make weight regulation more difficult:** Itziar Lamiquiz-Moneo et al., "Genetic Predictors of Weight Loss in Overweight and Obese Subjects," *Scientific Reports* 9 (2019): 10770, https://doi.org/10.1038/s41598-019-47283-5.

12 **can lead to changes:** Jérôme J. Heindel et al., "Obesity II: Establishing

Causal Links Between Chemical Exposures and Obesity," *Biochemical Pharmacology* 199 (2022): 115015, https://doi.org/10.1016/j.bcp.2022.115015.

12 affecting whether certain genes: Alicia Veiga-Lopez et al., "Obesogenic Endocrine Disrupting Chemicals: Identifying Knowledge Gaps," *Trends in Endocrinology & Metabolism* 29, no. 9 (2018): 607–25, https://doi.org/10.1016/j.tem.2018.06.003.

12 may experience different weight outcomes: Carmen M. Aguilera, Juan Olza, and Ángel Gil, "Genetic Susceptibility to Obesity and Metabolic Syndrome in Childhood," *Nutrición Hospitalaria* 28, suppl. 5 (2013): S44–S55, https://doi.org/10.3305/nh.2013.28.sup5.6917.

12 parents' weight at preconception: James R. Craig et al., "Obesity, Male Infertility, and the Sperm Epigenome," *Fertility and Sterility* 107, no. 4 (2017): 848–59, https://doi.org/10.1016/j.fertnstert.2017.02.115.

12 determine the weight of their future offspring: Marion Lecorguillé et al., "Impact of Parental Lifestyle Patterns in the Preconception and Pregnancy Periods on Childhood Obesity," *Frontiers in Nutrition* 10 (2023): 1166981, https://doi.org/10.3389/fnut.2023.1166981.

12 increasing the child's obesity risk: Melanie A. Schübel, Cornelia M. Prehn, and Dorothea Böhm, "Recent Developments on the Role of Epigenetics in Obesity and Metabolic Disease," *Clinical Epigenetics* 7 (2015): 66, https://doi.org/10.1186/s13148-015-0101-5.

12 A fetus exposed: Stephanie A. Bayol and Clare M. Reynolds, "Programming by Maternal Obesity: A Pathway to Poor Cardiometabolic Health in the Offspring," *Proceedings of the Nutrition Society* 81, no. 3 (2022): 227–42, https://doi.org/10.1017/S0029665122001914.

12 High consumption of ultraprocessed foods: Renata Liberali, Eliziane Kupek, and Mauro A. A. Assis, "Dietary Patterns and Childhood Obesity Risk: A Systematic Review," *Childhood Obesity* 16, no. 2 (2020): 70–85, https://doi.org/10.1089/chi.2019.0059.

12 Lack of key nutrients: Abílio Pereira and Elisa Keating, "Maternal Folate and Metabolic Programming of the Offspring: A Systematic Review of the Literature," *Reproductive Toxicology* 120 (2023): 108439, https://doi.org/10.1016/j.reprotox.2023.108439.

13 the body is more likely: Johannes A. M. J. L. Janssen, "Hyperinsulinemia and Its Pivotal Role in Aging, Obesity, Type 2 Diabetes, Cardiovascular Disease and Cancer," *International Journal of Molecular Sciences* 22, no. 15 (2021): 7797, https://doi.org/10.3390/ijms22157797.

13 **Conditions linked to insulin dysfunction:** Antonio A. da Silva et al., "Role of Hyperinsulinemia and Insulin Resistance in Hypertension: Metabolic Syndrome Revisited," *Canadian Journal of Cardiology* 36, no. 5 (2020): 671–82, https://doi.org/10.1016/j.cjca.2020.02.066.

13 **leading to increased hunger:** Nidia Martínez-Sánchez, "There and Back Again: Leptin Actions in White Adipose Tissue," *International Journal of Molecular Sciences* 21, no. 17 (2020): 6039, https://doi.org/10.3390/ijms21176039.

13 **leading to persistent hunger and overeating:** Susan M. Gray, Laura C. Page, and Jenny Tong, "Ghrelin Regulation of Glucose Metabolism," *Journal of Neuroendocrinology* 31, no. 7 (2019): e12705, https://doi.org/10.1111/jne.12705.

14 **contributes to central (abdominal) weight gain:** Rachel E. Van Pelt, Kathleen M. Gavin, and Wendy M. Kohrt, "Regulation of Body Composition and Bioenergetics by Estrogens," *Endocrinology and Metabolism Clinics of North America* 44, no. 3 (2015): 663–76, https://doi.org/10.1016/j.ecl.2015.05.011.

16 **leading to increased abdominal fat storage:** Paul A. Heine et al., "Increased Adipose Tissue in Male and Female Estrogen Receptor-Alpha Knockout Mice," *Proceedings of the National Academy of Sciences of the United States of America* 97, no. 23 (2000): 12729–34, https://doi.org/10.1073/pnas.97.23.12729.

16 **making weight management more challenging:** Benjamin M. Steiner and Daniel C. Berry, "The Regulation of Adipose Tissue Health by Estrogens," *Frontiers in Endocrinology* 13 (2022): 889923, https://doi.org/10.3389/fendo.2022.889923.

16 **a higher risk of developing:** Fatemeh Ebtekar, Saeid Dalvand, and Reza Ghanei Gheshlagh, "The Prevalence of Metabolic Syndrome in Postmenopausal Women: A Systematic Review and Meta-Analysis in Iran," *Diabetes & Metabolic Syndrome* 12, no. 6 (2018): 955–60, https://doi.org/10.1016/j.dsx.2018.06.002.

17 **leading to overeating and weight gain:** Karsten Ronit and Jeanette D. Jensen, "Obesity and Industry Self-Regulation of Food and Beverage Marketing: A Literature Review," *European Journal of Clinical Nutrition* 68, no. 7 (2014): 753–59, https://doi.org/10.1038/ejcn.2014.60.

17 **more than 50 percent:** "Ultraprocessed Foods Account for More than Half of Calories Consumed at Home," Johns Hopkins Bloomberg School of Public Health, December 10, 2024, https://publichealth.jhu

.edu/2024/ultraprocessed-foods-account-for-more-than-half-of-calories-consumed-at-home.

17 **making us crave more:** Ashley N. Gearhardt et al., "Social, Clinical, and Policy Implications of Ultra-Processed Food Addiction," *BMJ* 382 (2023): e072969, https://doi.org/10.1136/bmj-2023-072969.

17 **strongly linked to obesity in adulthood:** Vincent J. Felitti et al., "Relationship of Childhood Abuse and Household Dysfunction to Many of the Leading Causes of Death in Adults," *American Journal of Preventive Medicine* 14, no. 4 (1998): 245–58, https://doi.org/10.1016/S0749-3797(98)00017-8.

17 **particularly around the abdomen:** Ka Man Yam, Daniel T. L. Shek, and Rachel C. F. Sun, "The Association Between Childhood Trauma and Adiposity in Adulthood: A Meta-Analysis," *Obesity Reviews* 21, no. 4 (2020): e12908, https://doi.org/10.1111/obr.12908.

18 **can rewire the brain's reward system:** Erik Hemmingsson, "A New Model of the Role of Psychological and Emotional Distress in Promoting Obesity: Conceptual Review with Implications for Treatment and Prevention," *Obesity Reviews* 15, no. 9 (2014): 769–79, https://doi.org/10.1111/obr.12197.

18 **can shape our relationship with food:** Hemmingsson, "A New Model of the Role of Psychological and Emotional Distress in Promoting Obesity."

18 **not just emotionally but through epigenetic changes:** Rachel Yehuda et al., "Holocaust Exposure Induced Intergenerational Effects on FKBP5 Methylation," *Biological Psychiatry* 80, no. 5 (2016): 372–80, https://doi.org/10.1016/j.biopsych.2015.08.005.

18 **increasing fat storage over time:** Yam et al., "The Association Between Childhood Trauma and Adiposity in Adulthood."

19 **Endocrine-disrupting chemicals (EDCs):** Maria Dalamaga et al., "The Role of Endocrine Disruptors Bisphenols and Phthalates in Obesity: Current Evidence, Perspectives and Controversies," *International Journal of Molecular Sciences* 25, no. 1 (2024): 675, https://doi.org/10.3390/ijms25010675.

19 **disrupt your natural metabolic processes:** Jerrold J. Heindel et al., "Metabolism Disrupting Chemicals and Obesity," *Nature Reviews Endocrinology* 13, no. 8 (2017): 536–46, https://doi.org/10.1038/nrendo.2017.42.

19 **making weight gain more likely:** Ruth Naomi et al., "Bisphenol A (BPA) Leading to Obesity and Cardiovascular Complications: A Compilation of Current in Vivo Study," *International Journal of Molecular Sciences* 23, no. 6 (2022): 2969, https://doi.org/10.3390/ijms23062969.

19 **influencing obesity rates across generations:** Yuxuan Zhang et al., "Association Between Exposure to a Mixture of Phenols, Pesticides, and Phthalates and Obesity: Comparison of Three Statistical Models," *Environment International* 123 (2019): 325–36, https://doi.org/10.1016/j.envint.2018.11.076; Katherine Schafte and Selena Bruna, "The Influence of Intergenerational Trauma on Epigenetics and Obesity in Indigenous Populations: A Scoping Review," *Epigenetics* 18, no. 1 (2023): 2260218, https://doi.org/10.1080/15592294.2023.2260218.

19 **because of biological changes:** Ana L. Santos and Saurabh Sinha, "Obesity and Aging: Molecular Mechanisms and Therapeutic Approaches," *Ageing Research Reviews* 67 (2021), doi:10.1016/j.arr.2021.101268.

20 **decreases by approximately 1 to 2 percent:** Susan B. Roberts and George A. Dallal, "The Effect of Age on Energy Expenditure," *The American Journal of Clinical Nutrition* 62, no. 5 (1995): 1053S–1061S, https://doi.org/10.1093/ajcn/62.5.1053S.

20 **progressive muscle loss:** John A. Batsis and Dennis T. Villareal, "Sarcopenic Obesity in Older Adults: Aetiology, Epidemiology and Treatment Strategies," *Nature Reviews Endocrinology* 14, no. 9 (2018): 513–37, https://doi.org/10.1038/s41574-018-0062-9.

20 **adults lose 3 to 8 percent:** Elena Volpi et al., "Muscle Tissue Changes with Aging," *Current Opinion in Clinical Nutrition and Metabolic Care* 7, no. 4 (2004): 405–10, https://doi.org/10.1097/01.mco.0000134362.76653.b2.

Chapter 2

31 **he was able to isolate:** Benjamin L. Furman, "The Development of Byetta (Exenatide) from the Venom of the Gila Monster as an Anti-diabetic Agent," *Toxicon* 59, no. 4 (2012): 464–71, https://doi.org/10.1016/j.toxicon.2010.12.016.

32 **Byetta became the first:** Robert J. Meyer, Approval Letter for NDA 021773, Byetta (exenatide) Injection, Department of Health and Human Services, April 28, 2005, https://www.accessdata.fda.gov/drugsatfda_docs/nda/2005/021773_Byetta_approv.pdf.

33 **In 2010, Novo Nordisk introduced:** Curtis J. Rosebraugh, Approval Letter for NDA 022341, Victoza (liraglutide) Injection, Department of

Health and Human Services, January 25, 2010, https://www.accessdata.fda.gov/drugsatfda_docs/nda/2010/022341s000approv.pdf.

35 **Most of these are expected:** Eka Melson et al., "What Is the Pipeline for Future Medications for Obesity?," *International Journal of Obesity* 49 (2025): 433–51, https://doi.org/10.1038/s41366-024-01473-y.

41 **had higher mortality rates:** Zhiyong Cai, Yafang Yang, and Jianzhong Zhang, "Obesity Is Associated with Severe Disease and Mortality in Patients with Coronavirus Disease 2019 (COVID-19): A Meta-analysis," *BMC Public Health* 21, no. 1 (2021): 1505, https://doi.org/10.1186/s12889-021-11546-6.

43 **Some clinics are attempting:** Mads Hach et al., "Impact of Manufacturing Process and Compounding on Properties and Quality of Follow-On GLP-1 Polypeptide Drugs," *Pharmaceutical Research* 41, no. 10 (2024): 1991–2014, https://doi.org/10.1007/s11095-024-03771-6.

43 **Compounded GLP-1 medications:** "FDA's Concerns with Unapproved GLP-1 Drugs Used for Weight Loss," U.S. Food and Drug Administration, May 30, 2025, https://www.fda.gov/drugs/postmarket-drug-safety-information-patients-and-providers/fdas-concerns-unapproved-glp-1-drugs-used-weight-loss.

43 **some patients are still turning:** U.S. Food and Drug Administration, "FDA's Concerns with Unapproved GLP_1 Drugs Used for Weight Loss," FDA.gov. Content current as of July 29, 2025. https://www.fda.gov/drugs/postmarket-drug-safety-information-patients-and-providers/fdas-concerns-unapproved-glp-1-drugs-used-weight-loss.

50 **GLP-1 agonists may help improve:** Adam Blackman et al., "Effect of Liraglutide 3 0 mg in Individuals with Obesity and Moderate or Severe Obstructive Sleep Apnea: The SCALE Sleep Apnea Randomized Clinical Trial," *International Journal of Obesity* 40, no. 8 (2016): 1310–19, https://doi.org/10.1038/ijo.2016.52.

51 **reduce the risk of major cardiovascular events:** Steven P. Marso et al., "Liraglutide and Cardiovascular Outcomes in Type 2 Diabetes," *New England Journal of Medicine* 375 (2016): 311–22, https://doi.org/10.1056/NEJMoa1603827.

51 **GPL-1 agonists may improve brain health:** William Wang et al., "Associations of Semaglutide with First-Time Diagnosis of Alzheimer's Disease in Patients with Type 2 Diabetes: Target Trial Emulation Using Nationwide Real-World Data in the US," *Alzheimer's & Dementia* 20, no. 12 (2024), https://doi.org/10.1002/alz.14313; Christian Hölscher. "Brain Glucagon-like Peptide-1: Regulation of Energy Balance and Impact on Neurode-

generative Diseases," *British Journal of Pharmacology* 166, no. 1 (2012): 79–87, https://doi.org/10.1111/j.1476-5381.2011.01687.x.

51 **their ability to prevent or slow down:** Jeffrey L. Cummings et al., "Evoke and Evoke+: Design of Two Large-Scale, Double-Blind, Placebo-Controlled, Phase 3 Studies Evaluating Efficacy, Safety, and Tolerability of Semaglutide in Early-Stage Symptomatic Alzheimer's Disease," *Alzheimer's Research & Therapy* 17, no. 14 (2025), https://doi.org/10.1186/s13195-024-01666-7.

51 **their potential to treat addiction:** Mette K. Klausen et al., "The Role of Glucagon-like Peptide-1 (GLP-1) in Addictive Disorders," *British Journal of Pharmacology* 179, no. 4 (2022): 625–41, https://doi.org/10.1111/bph.15677; Nora D. Volkow and Rong Xu, "GLP-1R Agonist Medications for Addiction Treatment," *Addiction* 120, no. 2 (2025): 198–200, https://doi.org/10.1111/add.16626.

Chapter 3

58 **BMI is a deeply flawed:** William H. Dietz, *The Science, Strengths, and Limitations of Body Mass Index* (National Academies Press, 2021).

60 **The only absolute contraindication:** "Ozempic (semaglutide) Injection, for Subcutaneous Use," U.S. Food and Drug Administration, September 2023, https://www.accessdata.fda.gov/drugsatfda_docs/label/2023/209637s020s021lbl.pdf.

60 **MTC is associated:** Muhammad Yasir, Nasir J. Mulji, and Asher Kasi, "Multiple Endocrine Neoplasias Type 2," in *StatPearls*, updated August 14, 2023 (StatPearls Publishing, 2023), https://www.ncbi.nlm.nih.gov/books/NBK519054.

60 **Early mice studies showed:** Lotte W. Madsen et al., "GLP-1 Receptor Agonists and the Thyroid: C-Cell Effects in Mice Are Mediated via the GLP-1 Receptor and Not Associated with RET Activation," *Endocrinology* 153, no. 3 (2012): 1538–47, https://doi.org/10.1210/en.2011-1954.

62 **In real-world use, pancreatitis:** Matteo Monami et al., "Glucagon-like Peptide-1 Receptor Agonists and Acute Pancreatitis: A Meta-analysis of Randomized Clinical Trials," *Diabetes Research and Clinical Practice* 103, no. 2 (2014): 269–75, https://doi.org/10.1016/j.diabres.2013.12.049; Xiaojing Cai et al., "Risk of Acute Pancreatitis After Glucagon-like Peptide-1 Receptor Agonist Use in Patients with Type 2 Diabetes and History of Pancreatitis," *Diabetes Research and Clinical Practice* 206 (2024): 110587, https://doi.org/10.1016/j.diabres.2024.110587.

66 **your prepregnancy weight matters:** Ilaria Inzani and Susan E. Ozanne, "Programming by Maternal Obesity: A Pathway to Poor Cardiometabolic Health in the Offspring," *Proceedings of the Nutrition Society* 81, no. 3 (2022): 227–42, https://doi.org/10.1017/S0029665122001914.

66 **a better chance at lifelong good health:** Merve Denizli, Maria L. Capitano, and Kailee L. Kua, "Maternal Obesity and the Impact of Associated Early-Life Inflammation on Long-Term Health of Offspring," *Frontiers in Cellular and Infection Microbiology* 12 (2022): 940937, https://doi org/10.3389/fcimb.2022.940937.

66 **Fertility also tends to improve:** Christopher A. Service et al., "The Impact of Obesity and Metabolic Health on Male Fertility: A Systematic Review," *Fertility and Sterility* 120, no. 6 (2023): 1098–111, https://doi.org/10.1016/j.fertnstert.2023.10.017.

66 **help reduce inflammation:** Serife Kislal, Lauren L. Shook, and Andrea G. Edlow, "Perinatal Exposure to Maternal Obesity: Lasting Cardiometabolic Impact on Offspring," *Prenatal Diagnosis* 40, no. 9 (2020): 1109–25, https://doi.org/10.1002/pd.5784.

66 **especially in patients with conditions:** Lisa C. Cooney and Anuja Dokras, "Beyond Fertility: Polycystic Ovary Syndrome and Long-Term Health," *Fertility and Sterility* 110, no. 5 (2018): 794–809, https://doi.org/10.1016/j.fertnstert.2018.08.021.

66 **an equally negative impact on fertility:** Dimuthu Ameraturga, Amina Gebeh, and Angela Amoako, "Obesity and Male Infertility," *Best Practice & Research Clinical Obstetrics & Gynaecology* 90 (2023): 102393, https://doi.org/10.1016/j.bpobgyn.2023.102393.

67 **In one small study involving semaglutide:** Haya Diab et al., "Subcutaneous Semaglutide During Breastfeeding: Infant Safety Regarding Drug Transfer into Human Milk," *Nutrients* 16, no. 17 (2024): 2886, https://doi.org/10.3390/nu16172886.

67 **Another study found that GLP-1:** Dominique R. F. Muller et al., "Effects of GLP-1 Agonists and SGLT2 Inhibitors During Pregnancy and Lactation on Offspring Outcomes: A Systematic Review of the Evidence," *Frontiers in Endocrinology* 14 (2023): 1215356, https://doi.org/10.3389/fendo.2023.1215356.

67 **a loss of lean muscle mass:** Barbara Sternfeld et al., "Physical Activity and Changes in Weight and Waist Circumference in Midlife Women: Findings from the Study of Women's Health Across the Nation," *American Journal of Epidemiology* 160, no. 9 (2004): 912–22, https://doi.org/10.1093/aje/kwh299.

67 **accumulate, on average, 1.5 pounds:** Sternfeld et al., "Physical Activity and Changes in Weight."

69 **currently FDA approved:** "FDA Approves Weight Management Drug for Patients Aged 12 and Older," U.S. Food and Drug Administration, December 4, 2020, https://www.fda.gov/drugs/news-events-human-drugs/fda-approves-weight-management-drug-patients-aged-12-and-older.

73 **chronic, multifactorial medical condition:** "Obesity and Overweight," World Health Organization, May 7, 2025, https://www.who.int/news-room/fact-sheets/detail/obesity-and-overweight.

Chapter 4

77 **have advanced, targeted training:** Laura Alexander, "The Benefits of Obesity Medicine Certification," *American Journal of Lifestyle Medicine* 13, no. 2 (2019): 161–64, https://doi.org/10.1177/1559827618818041.

78 **just under 10,000 certified obesity medicine specialists:** American Board of Obesity Medicine, "More than 1,800 Achieve First-Time Obesity Medicine Certification," PRWeb, January 16, 2025, https://www.prweb.com/releases/more-than-1-800-achieve-first-time-obesity-medicine-certification-302352852.html.

78 **fastest-growing medical specialty:** Ted Kyle, "Why Is Obesity Medicine the Fastest Growing Medical Specialty in the US?," *Patient Care Online*, April 22, 2020, https://www.patientcareonline.com/view/why-is-obesity-medicine-the-fastest-growing-medical-specialty-in-the-us.

84 **signal a red flag when offered routinely:** "Compounding Risk Alerts," U.S. Food and Drug Administration, updated April 24, 2025, https://www.fda.gov/drugs/human-drug-compounding/compounding-risk-alerts.

94 **likely spend less on food:** "Could Obesity Drugs Take a Bite Out of the Food Industry?," Morgan Stanley, September 5, 2023, https://www.morganstanley.com/ideas/obesity-drugs-food-industry.

94 **offer significant savings:** "Savings Card, Cost & Coverage Support | Zepbound® (tirzepatide)," Eli Lilly and Company, accessed April 30, 2025, https://www.zepbound.lilly.com/savings-support; "Our Medicines: Diabetes Medications," Novo Nordisk, accessed April 30, 2025, https://zepbound.lilly.com/coverage-savings.

97 **These are more rigorously regulated:** "Information for Outsourcing Facilities," U.S. Food and Drug Administration, March 29, 2022, https://www.fda.gov/drugs/human-drug-compounding/information-outsourcing-facilities.

97 **legally compounded medication must differ:** "Current Good Manufacturing Practice—Guidance for Human Drug Compounding Outsourcing Facilities Under Section 503B of the FD&C Act Guidance for Industry," U.S. Food and Drug Administration, January 2020, https://www.fda.gov/regulatory-information/search-fda-guidance-documents/current-good-manufacturing-practice-guidance-human-drug-compounding-outsourcing-facilities-under.

Chapter 5

108 **their blood pressure may improve:** Feng Sun et al., "Impact of GLP-1 Receptor Agonists on Blood Pressure, Heart Rate and Hypertension Among Patients with Type 2 Diabetes: A Systematic Review and Network Meta-analysis," *Diabetes Research and Clinical Practice* 110 (2015): 26–37, https://doi.org/10.1016/j.diabres.2015.07.007.

113 **potential treatments for alcohol dependency:** Christian S. Hendershot et al., "Use of GLP-1 Receptor Agonists to Treat Substance and Alcohol Use Disorders Is Promising but Premature," UNC Health, December 5, 2023, https://news.unchealthcare.org/2023/12/use-of-glp-1-receptor-agonists-to-treat-substance-and-alcohol-use-disorders-is-promising-but-premature/.

124 **The scales with the most accurate readings:** Minseon Kim and Hyuntae Kim, "Accuracy of Segmental Multi-frequency Bioelectrical Impedance Analysis for Assessing Whole-Body and Appendicular Fat Mass and Lean Soft Tissue Mass in Frail Women Aged 75 Years and Older," *European Journal of Clinical Nutrition* 67, no. 4 (2013): 395–400, https://doi.org/10.1038/ejcn.2013.39.

Chapter 6

130 **Whenever skeletal muscle contracts:** Bianca E. M. Zunner et al., "Myokines and Resistance Training: A Narrative Review," *International Journal of Molecular Sciences* 23, no. 7 (2022): 3501, https://doi.org/10.3390/ijms23073501; Marta Gomarasca, Giuseppe Banfi, and Giovanni Lombardi, "Myokines: The Endocrine Coupling of Skeletal Muscle and Bone," *Advances in Clinical Chemistry* 94 (2020): 155–218, https://doi.org/10.1016/bs.acc.2019.07.010.

130 **Myokines have positive effects:** Ying Ren et al., "Adipokines, Hepatokines and Myokines: Focus on Their Role and Molecular Mechanisms in Adipose Tissue Inflammation," *Frontiers in Endocrinology* 13 (2022): 873699, https://doi.org/10.3389/fendo.2022.873699; Christine Hoffmann and Cora Weigert, "Skeletal Muscle as an Endocrine Organ:

The Role of Myokines in Exercise Adaptations," *Cold Spring Harbor Perspectives in Medicine* 7, no. 11 (2017): a029793, https://doi.org/10.1101/cshperspect.a029793.

130 **It even helps stabilize:** Sze-Xian Sui et al., "Skeletal Muscle Health and Cognitive Function: A Narrative Review," *International Journal of Molecular Sciences* 22, no. 1 (2020): 255, https://doi.org/10.3390/ijms22010255.

131 **The more muscle mass you have:** Hiroki Nishikawa et al., "Metabolic Syndrome and Sarcopenia," *Nutrients* 13, no. 10 (2021): 3519, https://doi.org/10.3390/nu13103519.

131 **researchers are starting to connect:** Seung Yoon Park, Byoung Ok Hwang, and Nam Yong Song, "The Role of Myokines in Cancer: Crosstalk Between Skeletal Muscle and Tumor," *BMB Reports* 56, no. 7 (July 2023): 365–73, https://doi.org/10.5483/BMBRep.2023-0064.

131 **has an anti-inflammatory effect:** L. V. Kapilevich et al., "Secretory Function of Skeletal Muscles: Producing Mechanisms and Myokines Physiological Effects" (in Russian), *Uspekhi Fiziologicheskikh Nauk* 47, no. 2 (2016): 7–26.

131 **Early studies even suggest:** Rudy Vangoitsenhoven, Chantal Mathieu, and Bart Van der Schueren, "GLP1 and Cancer: Friend or Foe?," *Endocrine-Related Cancer* 19, no. 5 (2012): F77–F88, https://doi.org/10.1530/ERC-12-0111.

132 **will affect your muscle mass:** Darcy L. Johannsen et al., "Effect of Weight Loss on Muscle Mass, Strength, and Aerobic Capacity," *Medicine & Science in Sports & Exercise* 48, no. 3 (2016): 499–508, https://doi.org/10.1249/MSS.0000000000001074.

134 **the highest thermic effect:** Monica Calcagno et al., "The Thermic Effect of Food: A Review," *Journal of the American College of Nutrition* 38, no. 6 (2019): 547–51, https://doi.org/10.1080/07315724.2018.1552544.

134 **The United States Department of Agriculture (USDA) recommends:** U.S. Department of Agriculture and U.S. Department of Health and Human Services, *Dietary Guidelines for Americans, 2020–2025*, 9th ed., December 2020, https://www.dietaryguidelines.gov/sites/default/files/2021-03/Dietary_Guidelines_for_Americans-2020-2025.pdf.

134 **International Society of Sports Nutrition:** Ralf Jäger et al., "Interna-

tional Society of Sports Nutrition Position Stand: Protein and Exercise," *Journal of the International Society of Sports Nutrition* 14, no. 1 (2017): 20, https://doi.org/10.1186/s12970-017-0177-8.

134 **European Society for Clinical Nutrition and Metabolism:** Nicolaas E. P. Deutz et al., "Protein Intake and Exercise for Optimal Muscle Function with Aging: Recommendations from the ESPEN Expert Group," *Clinical Nutrition* 33, no. 6 (2014): 929–36, https://doi.org/10.1016/j.clnu.2014.04.007.

134 **They are published:** Stuart M. Phillips and Luc J. C. van Loon, "Dietary Protein for Athletes: From Requirements to Optimum Adaptation," *The American Journal of Clinical Nutrition* 101, no. 6 (2015): 1320S–1328S, https://doi.org/10.3945/ajcn.114.084038.

135 **amino acids make up proteins:** "Amino Acids," Cleveland Clinic, accessed June 7, 2025, https://my.clevelandclinic.org/health/articles/22243-amino-acids.

138 **Research shows that 30 grams:** Jose L. Areta et al., "Timing and Distribution of Protein Ingestion During Prolonged Recovery from Resistance Exercise Alters Myofibrillar Protein Synthesis," *Journal of Physiology* 591, no. 9 (2013): 2319–31, https://doi.org/10.1113/jphysiol.2012.244897.

149 **cause microscopic damage to them:** Felipe Damas et al., "The Development of Skeletal Muscle Hypertrophy Through Resistance Training: The Role of Muscle Damage and Muscle Protein Synthesis," *European Journal of Applied Physiology* 118, no. 3 (2018): 485–500, https://doi.org/10.1007/s00421-017-3792-9.

151 **your body can't rebuild:** Murilo Dáttilo et al., "Effects of Sleep Deprivation on Acute Skeletal Muscle Recovery After Exercise," *Medicine & Science in Sports & Exercise* 52, no. 2 (2020): 507–14, https://doi.org/10.1249/MSS.0000000000002137.

Chapter 7

161 **The appetite suppression should feel consistent:** Megan J. Dailey and Timothy H. Moran, "Glucagon-like Peptide 1 and Appetite," *Trends in Endocrinology and Metabolism* 24, no. 2 (2013): 85–91, https://doi.org/10.1016/j.tem.2012.11.008.

165 **Rare monogenic mutations:** Ruth J. F. Loos and Giles S. H. Yeo, "The Genetics of Obesity: From Discovery to Biology," *Nature Reviews Ge-*

netics 23, no. 2 (2022): 120–33, https://doi.org/10.1038/s41576-021-00414-z.

176 **This warning is based:** Lars Wichmann Madsen et al., "GLP-1 Receptor Agonists and the Thyroid: C-Cell Effects in Mice Are Mediated via the GLP-1 Receptor and Not Associated with RET Activation," *Endocrinology* 153, no. 3 (2012): 1538–47, https://doi.org/10.1210/en.2011-1864.

Index

A
acid reflux, 46, 171–72
active ingredients
  basic facts about, 89
  liraglutide, 91
  semaglutide, 90
  tirzepatide, 91
addiction, 51
adults, percent of, with obesity in United States, 5–6
adverse childhood experiences (ACEs), 17
aging
  muscle loss and, 20, 72
  weight gain and, 19–21
air travel with GLP-1 medications, 118
alcohol, 71, 112–13
American Board of Obesity Medicine website, 80
The American Journal of Clinical Nutrition, 134
American Medical Association (AMA), 9
amino acids, 135–36
Amylin Pharmaceuticals, 32
antidepressants, 21–22

appetite suppression
  dosage and, 159, 160, 161
  excessive, 166–67
  food noise and, 109
  nausea and, 162
  treatment starting day and, 116
at-home body composition scale, monitoring with progress, 123–24
autoimmune conditions, medications for, 22

B
Bimagrumab, 36
blood pressure, medications for, 22
body composition
  analysis and ideal weight, 106
  information obtained from scans, 121–23
  metrics for obesity, 25–26
  monitoring with at-home scale, 123–24
  protein intake and, 164
  tapering off medication and, 194–95
  temperature regulation and, 68
  types of scans, 120–21

Index

body impedance analysis (BIA), 120–21
body mass index (BMI)
  FDA approval for GLP-1 medications and, 58
  insurance companies' approval for GLP-1 medications, 58–59
  obesity or overweight diagnosis and, 24–25
brain
  action of GLP-1 medications in, 38
  health of, and GLP-1 medications, 51
  reward system in, 11
breast changes, 209–10
breastfeeding, 67
Bydureon, 33, 37
Byetta, 32–33, 37, 41

C

CagriSema, 35
caloric intake and fat storage, 38
cancer
  GLP-1 medications and, 131–32
  medullary thyroid carcinoma, 60, 61, 176
  muscle mass, metabolic health, and treatment for, 131
  progression of, 51
cardiac muscle, 130
character flaw, as cause of obesity, xiii, 3, 4–5, 7
children
  diet during early years, 12
  eligibility of, for GLP-1, 69–70
  percent of, with obesity in United States, 5–6

chronic diseases. *See specific diseases*
chronic diseases linked to obesity, 6, 9
cold sensitivity, 204–6
college students, 70–71
compounded medications
  choosing pharmacy, 97
  described, 42–44
  questions to ask about, 97–98
  risks, 96
constipation, 170
cortisol and fat storage, 13
costs, 93–95, 191–92
  See also eligibility for GLP-1; preexisting conditions and eligibility
covid-19 pandemic, 41
Cushing's syndrome/disease, 15

D

dehydration, 46, 171
diabetes
  gestational, 15–16
  type 1, 61, 63
  See also type 2 diabetes
diagnosis, 24–27, 92
diarrhea, 170
dieting and GLP-1 medications, 38
digestive changes, 46
direct-to-patient pharmacy delivery programs, 95
diseases, 9
  See also specific diseases
dosage of GLP-1 medications
  appetite suppression and, 159, 160, 161
  decreasing, 161–63, 187–89

factors influencing maintenance, 189–92
goal when setting, 72–73
increasing, 161
liraglutide (Saxenda and Victoza), 91
making most of each, 159
microdoses, 192–93
muscle mass and, 190–91
pausing decrease in, 189
semaglutide (Wegovy and Ozempic), 90, 160–61
side effects and, 168
starting, 104, 106
therapeutic, 92
tirzepatide (Zepbound and Mounjaro), 91
titration timelines, 106–8
weight loss and, 158, 160–61, 163
dual-energy X-ray absorptiometry (DEXA) scan, 120

E
eligibility for GLP-1
breastfeeding, 67
children, 69–70
FDA approved categories, 58
insurance companies and, 58–59
older adults, 20, 71–72
perimenopause and menopause, 67–68
pregnancy, 66–67
young adults, 70–71
See also preexisting conditions and eligibility
Eli Lilly and Company, 32, 34, 35
emotional issues, 18
endocrine-disrupting chemicals (EDCs), 19
endocrinology, 77–78, 80
Eng, John, xv, 30–31
environment and weight gain
adverse childhood experiences, 17
emotional issues, 18
endocrine-disrupting chemicals (EDCs), 19
epigenetics, 12
factors contributing to, 6
generational trauma, 18
long-term marginalization, 18
overconsumption, 16–17
sedentary lifestyle, 19
ultraprocessed foods, 6, 12, 17
epigenetics, 12
estrogen
decrease in menopause and perimenopause, 16
fat storage locations, 14
European Society for Clinical Nutrition and Metabolism (ESPEN), 134
exendin-4, 31, 32
exercise, individual's relationship with, 56
"expiration effect," 116

F
facial volume, loss of, 207–8
family history of obesity, 11
fat
distribution in body of, 123
lowering percentage of body, 102
muscle and, 131

fat – *cont.*
  regulation of internal temperature and, 204–5
  temperature regulation and, 68
  visceral, 102, 120
fatigue, 46, 174
fat oxidation, 38
fat storage
  caloric intake versus use and, 38
  cortisol and, 13
  estrogen and locations of, 14
  insulin resistance and, 14
FDA approval of GLP-1 medications
  for chronic weight management, 34, 90, 91
  clinical criteria, 58
  for obesity, 42
  for obesity or overweight with at least one weight-related comorbidity, 58
  for type 2 diabetes, 58, 90, 91
FDA approval of non-GLP-1 weight loss medications, 47–48
FDA approval process, 44
fetal development, 12
503A pharmacies, 97
503B outsourcing facilities, 97
follow-up visits
  checklist of topics to cover, 119, 232–33
  choosing provider and, 83, 88
  importance of, 119
  missing, 201
  during weight maintenance, 199–200

food
  building new routines with, 114–15
  designed to create cravings, 110
  eating out, 115
  GLP-1 and, habits, 114
  GLP-1 and enjoyment of, 111–12
  grams of protein in common, 229
  relationship with, 56, 57, 191
  return of hunger, 167
  rewiring relationship with, 110, 196, 197
food noise
  appetite suppression and, 109
  described, 57
  "mental quieting" of, 39
foot changes, 208–9

G
gallbladder issues, 175–76
gallbladder removal, 61
gas, 170–71
generational trauma, 18
genetics, 11–12
gestational diabetes, 15–16
ghrelin, 13, 38
GIP (glucagon-inhibiting protein), 34–35, 40
GLP-1 (hormone), 14, 30, 34–35, 38, 40
GLP-1 (natural hormone), 38, 48–49
GLP-1 medications (receptor agonists)
  action of, 38
  administration of, 41–42
  benefits of, beyond weight loss, 50–51

cancer and, 131–32
combining other drugs
   with, 165
compounded, 96–98
as control not cure, 183
development of, 29, 30–34, 37
dieting and, 38
differences among, 88–89
evaluating, 49
GLP-1 receptors in brain and, 39
inflammation and, 51
long-acting nature of, 160
mechanism of, 14, 38–39
number of, on market, 89
oral, 36
Ozempic as poster child of, 34
in pipeline, 35–36
potential of, for society, 224–25
reasons for current awareness
   of, 41–42
sharing experience with
   others, 217–18
stopping abruptly, 194
traditional weight loss drugs
   compared to, 46–47
transporting, 118
treatment length, 49, 72–73
GLP-1 receptors in brain, 39
goals, setting correct, 102
GPS system
   importance of, 127–28
   maintenance of muscle-preserving
      habits, 129–33
   progress using, 155
   protein in. *See* protein
   strength training. *See* strength
      training

H
Habener, Joel, 30
hair thinning/shedding, 173
Haver, Mary Claire, xi–xii
headaches, 46, 173
heart attacks, 51
heartburn, 46
holidays, 198
hormone replacement therapy,
   61, 68
hormones
   body temperature regulation
      and, 205
   cortisol, 13
   estrogen, 14, 16
   ghrelin, 13, 38
   GIP, 34–35, 40
   GLP-1, 14, 30, 34–35, 38, 40
   GLP-1 medications and, 38–39
   incretins, 35, 37
   insulin, 13, 33–34, 102
   leptin, 13
   peptide YY (PYY), 14, 38
   retatrutide, 35, 37, 40
   testosterone, 14, 15
   thyroid, 14, 20
   weight gain and, 13, 14–16
hypertension, 58
hypothyroidism, 14, 15

I
incretins, basic facts about, 35
infancy, diet during, 12
inflammation
   GLP-1 medications and, 51
   medications for, 22
   muscle and, 131, 193

injections
  changing day of, 117
  mastering, 117–18
  reactions requiring immediate medical attention, 118
  start date for, 116–17
  storing and transporting medications for, 118
insulin
  liraglutide and stimulation of, 33–34
  role of, 13
  visceral fat and, 102
insulin resistance
  conditions linked to, 13
  described, 14
  fat storage and, 14
  in pregnancy, 15–16
insurance companies
  eligibility for GLP-1 and, 58–59
  navigating coverage, 95
International Society of Sports Nutrition (ISSN), 134
irritable bowel syndrome (IBS), 61, 62–63

K
kidney function, 72

L
leptin, 13
life after weight loss: physical adjustments
  breast changes, 209–10
  cold sensitivity, 204–6
  excess skin, 174, 206–7
  feet changes, 208–9
  loss of facial volume, 207–8
  sleep changes, 210–11
life after weight loss: psychological adjustments
  judging eating habits or bodies of others, 216
  letting go of former mindset, 220
  self-perception changes needed, 212
  sharing experience with others and, 218
  therapy for, 212–13
  unexpected, 211
life after weight loss: social adjustments
  confronting weight stigma, 215–16
  handling negative comments, 214
  scripts for social situations, 215
  unexpected reactions of others, 213–14
lifestyle
  changes to achieve protein intake goals, 144–46
  changes to get most out of GLP-1 medications. *See* GPS system
  epigenetics and, 12
  patterns and weight gain, 23–24
  sedentary, 19
  tapering off medication and, 194
  ultraprocessed foods, 6, 12, 17
liraglutide
  basic facts about, 91–92
  dosage, 91
  FDA approval of, 42
  insulin stimulation and, 33–34
  titration, 108
  weight loss and, 34

M

magnetic resonance imaging (MRI) scan, 120
manufacturer coupons, 94–95
marginalization, long-term, 18
MariTide, 36
MC4R mutations, 165–66
medications and weight gain, 21–22
medullary thyroid carcinoma (MTC), 60, 51, 176
menopause
  estrogen decrease in, 16
  GLP-1 medications during, 67–68
metabolic syndrome, 13
metabolism
  aging and changes in, 19–22
  markers of healthy, 26
  muscles and, 102–3
  response to GLP-1 medications and, 165
  skeletal muscle and, 130
  treatment for cancer and, 131
microdosing, 192–93
Mojsov, Svetlana, 30
Monlunabant, 36
mood stabilizers, 21–22
moral failings, as cause of obesity, xiii, 3, 4–5, 7
Mounjaro
  FDA approval of, 42, 91
  See also tirzepatide
multifactorial chronic diseases, obesity recognized as one, 9
multiple endocrine neoplasia type 2 (MEN2), 60, 61
muscle memory, 153
muscle(s)
  complete protein and, 135, 136
  exercises to help with sagging skin, 174, 207
  fat and, 131
  GPS system and, 129–33
  heat generation by, 205
  loss and aging, 20, 72
  loss and dosage, 159, 162
  loss and GLP-1 medications, 132
  loss as percent of overall weight loss, 105
  loss as secondary side effect, 173
  mass and maintenance of GLP-1 medications dosage, 190–91
  mass and weight maintenance, 196–97
  mass by body segment, 123
  metabolism and, 102–3
  protein and, 133–34, 135, 136, 140–41, 153, 205
  strength training and, 149–50
  treatment for cancer and, 131
  types of, 130, 193
myokines, 130, 131

N

nausea, 46, 162, 169–70
Novo Nordisk, 33

O

obesity
  adults in United States with, 5–6
  BMI and, 24–25
  children in United States with, 5–6
  as chronic condition, 184–85
  chronic diseases linked to, 6

obesity – *cont.*
  covid-19 patients and, 41
  defined, 5
  diagnosing, 24–27
  failure to understand as medical condition, xiii, 4–5, 7
  family history of, 11
  FDA approval of GLP-1 medications for, 42, 58
  global increase in, 5–6
  as lifelong struggle, 56–57, 73
  previous ideas about cause of, xiii, 3, 4–5, 7
  recognized as chronic, multifactorial disease, 9
  sudden shift in life as cause of, 57, 73
  treatment of symptoms of, 7–8
obesity medicine as specialty, 77–78, 80
obstructive sleep apnea, 50, 58, 210
off-label uses, 69, 191–92, 193
older adults, 20, 71–72
Orforglipron, 35
osteoarthritis, 58
overweight
  BMI and, 24–25
  causes of. *See* weight gain, causes of
  diagnosing, 24–27
  FDA approval of GLP-1 medications for, with at least one weight-related comorbidity, 58
  as lifelong struggle, 56–57, 73
  predisposition to, as chronic, 185
  sudden shift in life as cause of becoming, 57, 73

Ozempic
  FDA approval of, 42, 90
  as poster child of GLP-1s, 34
  See also semaglutide
"Ozempic face," 207–8

P
pancreatic enzymes, elevated, 61
pancreatitis, 61–62, 174–75
peptide YY (PYY)
  effect of GLP-1 on, 38
  satiety feelings and, 14
perimenopause
  estrogen decrease in, 16
  GLP-1 medications during, 67–68
plant-based diets, 136–37
polycystic ovarian syndrome (PCOS)
  basic facts about, 14–15
  GLP-1 medications and, 61, 64–65
POMC mutations, 165–66
postpartum weight retention/gain, 16
prediabetes
  GLP-1 medications approval, 58
  insulin dysfunction and, 13
preexisting conditions and eligibility categories, 60
  elevated pancreatic enzymes, 61
  gallbladder removal, 61
  hormone replacement therapy, 61
  hypertension, 58
  irritable bowel syndrome, 61, 62–63
  pancreatitis, 61–62
  polycystic ovarian syndrome, 61, 64
  prediabetes, 58
  sleep apnea, 58
  thyroid conditions, 60–61
  type 1 diabetes, 61, 63

pregnancy
  excess weight gained
    during, 16
  GLP-1 medications during,
    66–67
  insulin resistance in, 15–16
progress
  GPS and, 155
  monitoring with at-home body
    composition scale, 123–24
  patience required, 177
  signs of, 104–5, 108–9
  tracking without body
    composition scale, 125
  weight plateaus and, 163–66
protein
  ability of body to absorb, 138
  amount needed, 134
  choosing protein powder, 140
  complete, 135–37
  dosage and, 160, 162–63
  excess skin and, 174, 207
  importance of, 132, 133–34
  intake and body composition,
    164
  loss of facial volume and, 208
  muscle and, 133–34, 135, 136,
    140–41, 153, 205
protein intake goals
  examples of meals to achieve,
    141–44
  game plan for managing, 228
  grams of protein in common
    foods, 229
  guidelines for achieving, 138–39
  lifestyle changes to
    achieve, 144–46

providers, choosing right
  ability to change and, 88
  board certification, 80
  custom treatment plan, 87
  diagnostic metrics used, 82
  experience prescribing GLP-1
    medications, 82
  first appointment, 81, 85–87,
    230–31
  follow-up visits and, 83, 88
  insurance coverage and, 85
  laboratory tests, 87
  specialties, 77–78
  telehealth platforms, 84–85

Q
Qsymia, 165

R
resistance training. *See* strength
  training
resting rate of caloric burn, 11
retatrutide, 35, 37, 40
Rybelsus, 36

S
Salas-Whalen, Rocio, basic
  facts about, xi, xiv–xv,
  xvi, 148–49
sarcopenia, 20, 72
satiety
  blunting of response, 11
  GLP-1 and feelings of, 14, 38, 110
  PYY and feelings of, 14
Saxenda
  FDA approval of, 34, 42, 91
  See also liraglutide

semaglutide
  basic facts about, 90
  compounded, 42–44
  development of, 34
  dosage, 90, 160–61
  FDA approval of, 42
  nausea and, 169
  oral, 36
  pen injection technique, 117
  titration, 90, 106–7
side effects of GLP-1 medications
  acid reflux, 46, 171–72
  common, 168–72
  constipation, 170
  dehydration, 46, 171
  diarrhea, 170
  digestive changes, 46
  fatigue, 46, 174
  gas, 170–71
  headaches, 46, 173
  heartburn, 46
  increase in dosage and, 159
  listening to body and, 177
  nausea, 46, 162, 169–70
  pancreatitis, 62
  proper use and, 45
  secondary, 173–74
  of semaglutide, 90
  start date and, 116
  titration and, 92, 162
  uncommon, 174–76
  vomiting, 172
skeletal muscle, 130, 193
skin, loose or sagging, 174, 206–7
sleep, 23, 150–51, 210–11
sleep apnea, 50, 58, 210
smooth muscle, 130

start date considerations, 116–17
storing GLP-1 medications, 118
strength training
  about, 147
  breast changes after
    weight loss, 209
  importance of, 146–47, 149
  injury prevention during, 151–53
  muscle and, 149–50
  muscle memory and, 153
  rest between workouts, 151
  typical workout, 147–48
  weights and repetitions, 147
stress
  from emotional issues, 18
  exposure of previous
    generations to, 12
  from long-term marginalization, 18
strokes, 51
Survodutide, 35

T
tapering off medication process, 188, 194–95
teenagers, 70–71
telehealth platforms, using, 84–85
testosterone, 14, 15
thyroid conditions, 60–61, 176
thyroid hormones (T3 and T4), 14, 20
tiredness, 46, 174
tirzepatide
  basic facts about, 91
  development of, 34
  dosage, 91
  FDA approval of, 42, 91
  management of blood sugar and
    metabolism by, 40

as mimicker of both GLP-1 and
     GIP hormones, 34, 40
  nausea and, 169
  titration, 107
titration
  decreasing dosage, 161–63,
     187–89, 194–95
  described, 90, 157
  factors influencing maintenance
     dose, 189–92
  fine-tuning, 158–61
  increasing dosage, 161
  of liraglutide, 108
  pausing decrease, 189
  of semaglutide, 90, 106–7
  side effects and, 92, 162
  of tirzepatide, 107
  See also dosage
transgenerational trauma, 12
transporting GLP-1 medications, 118
treatment of symptoms of obesity, 7–8
type 1 diabetes, 61, 63
type 2 diabetes
  FDA approval of GLP-1
     medications for, 58, 90, 91
  GLP-1 medications development
     and, 29, 32
  insulin dysfunction and, 13
  medications for, 22
  seriousness of, xv

U
ultraprocessed foods
  accessibility and affordability of, 6
  basic facts about, 17
  consumption of, in infancy and
     early childhood, 12

United States, increase in
     obesity in, 5–6

V
vacations, 198–99
Victoza
  development of, 33
  FDA approval of, 42, 91
  See also liraglutide
visceral fat, 102, 120
vomiting, 172

W
Wegovy
  FDA approval of, 42, 90
  See also semaglutide
weight
  FDA approval of chronic weight
     management GLP-1 medications,
     90, 91
  gain and hormones, 13, 14–16
  ideal, 106
  microdosing, 192–93
  predisposition to gain, as
     chronic, 185
  regaining, 200–202
  See also environment and weight
     gain; weight gain, causes of
weight gain, causes of
  environmental, 16–19
  genes and epigenetic
     changes, 11–12
  hormonal, 13–16
  life stages, 15–16, 19–21
  lifestyle patterns, 23–24
  medications, 21–22
  previous ideas about, xiii, 3, 4–5, 7

weight loss
- genetic mutations and, 165–66
- GLP-1 medications dosage and, 158, 160–61, 163
- goal amount, 59
- liraglutide and, 34
- muscle loss as part of overall, 105, 132
- pace of, 103
- rate of, 48, 105
- sustainable, 104

weight loss medications, non-GLP-1
- FDA approval of, 47–48
- GLP-1 medications compared to, 46–47
- mechanisms of, 47–48

weight maintenance
- appetite and, 195–96
- continuing GLP-1 medications for, 183–86
- decreasing dosage, 187–89
- factors influencing, 189–92
- follow-up visits during, 199–200
- holidays and, 198
- mindset during, 182–83
- muscle and, 196–97
- vacations and, 198–99

weight plateaus, 163–66
whey protein, 135
willpower problems, as cause of obesity, xiii, 3, 4–5, 7
World Health Organization (WHO), 5, 9

Y

Young, Andrew, 32
young adults, 70–71

Z

Zepbound
- FDA approval of, 42, 91
- injection site irritation and, 117–18
- *See also* tirzepatide

About the Author

Dr. Rocio Salas-Whalen is a board-certified endocrinologist specializing in obesity medicine, women's hormonal health, and metabolic care. As one of the earliest physicians in the United States to adopt GLP-1 medications in clinical practice, she has helped thousands of patients reclaim their health with science-backed, compassionate care.

Born and raised in Mexico, Dr. Salas-Whalen immigrated to the United States at age twenty-five to pursue her lifelong dream of becoming a physician. Today, she leads a thriving private practice in New York City, where she combines cutting-edge medicine with empathy, empowerment, and a fierce commitment to her patients' well-being.

Her work has been featured on Univision, the Mel Robbins Podcast, and international medical conferences. Known for her no-nonsense approach to weight loss, hormone therapy, and the stigma surrounding obesity, she is a trusted voice for patients who have been dismissed, overlooked, or told to "try harder."

This book is the guide she wishes her patients who use GLP-1s had from the very beginning: the science, the mindset, and the hope of finally breaking free from the cycle of dieting and stepping into lasting change.

nyendocrinology.com
Instagram: @drsalaswhalen
TikTok: @newyorkendocrinology